Medical Insurance Eligibility Verification

-

The Comprehensive Guide

by

VIRUTI SHIVAN

Masters in Clinical Psychology (Major)

"In books, as in life, it's not the size or looks but the content that matters."

Disclaimer: *The information in this book is for general information purposes only and is not professional advice. It's not a replacement for proper training, diagnosis, treatment, or guidance from qualified professionals. Although we've tried to ensure accuracy, there may be errors or omissions, so it's essential to consult experts in the relevant fields and independently verify information when needed.*

Introduction

Welcome to the fascinating world of Medical Insurance Eligibility Verification! Imagine you're embarking on a thrilling adventure, one where the mysteries of healthcare insurance are unraveled, and the secrets of navigating this complex system are revealed. This journey is not just for the healthcare professionals but for anyone intrigued by the intricacies of medical insurance.

Why is This Important?

In the grand theater of healthcare, insurance eligibility verification plays a leading role. It's the art of ensuring that patients' insurance coverage aligns with the medical services they seek. This may sound simple, but it's as intricate as a masterfully woven tapestry. Every thread counts, and missing even one can lead to a cascade of billing mishaps, frustrated patients, and lost revenue.

A Glimpse into the Adventure Ahead

As we delve into this guide, we're not just going to skim the surface. Oh no, we're diving deep! We'll start by laying the foundation, understanding the basics of health insurance – think of it as learning the rules of the game. Then, we'll maneuver through the steps of the verification process, unraveling the complexities with the finesse of a skilled detective.

We'll tackle the tricky lingo of insurance, making sense of those perplexing terms that often sound like a foreign language. Next, we're going to explore the role of technology – our trusty sidekick in this adventure – and see how it's revolutionizing the insurance verification process.

But what's a quest without some challenges? We'll face them head-on, from understanding legal and regulatory aspects to navigating different healthcare settings. We'll also learn how to manage patient expectations and experience, ensuring that this journey is as smooth as possible for those who matter most – the patients.

In the heart of this journey, we'll focus on the people who make it all happen – the healthcare professionals. We'll dive into the world of training, development, and the importance of continuous learning. And because no man is an island, we'll look at the power of networking and how it can foster professional growth.

Finally, we'll gaze into the crystal ball, contemplating the future of insurance verification. We'll ponder over upcoming trends and how to stay ahead in this ever-evolving landscape.

Embark on This Journey with Us

So, buckle up! Whether you're a seasoned professional or a curious novice, this guide promises to be an enlightening expedition through the world of medical insurance eligibility verification. Let's turn the page and begin this exciting adventure together!

Chapter 1: The Basics of Medical Insurance Eligibility Verification

1.1 Understanding Health Insurance Concepts

Imagine you're at the start of a maze – the maze of health insurance. To navigate it successfully, you first need to understand its layout. This is what we're doing in this section – getting a grip on the basic concepts of health insurance, the foundation upon which everything else in this maze is built.

What is Health Insurance?

Health insurance is like a safety net, designed to protect individuals from the high costs of medical care. It's an agreement where individuals or their employers pay a premium, and in return, the insurance company agrees to cover a portion of their medical expenses.

Types of Health Insurance Plans

There are several types of health insurance plans, each with its quirks:

- **HMO (Health Maintenance Organization):** Think of it as a tight-knit community. You have a primary care physician (PCP) who coordinates all your care and refers you to specialists within a specific network.

- **PPO (Preferred Provider Organization):** This is more like having a VIP pass. You have more freedom to choose your healthcare providers and don't need referrals for specialists. However, staying within the network gets you better rates.

- **EPO (Exclusive Provider Organization):** A blend of HMO and PPO. You have the liberty to see any provider within the network without referrals, but out-of-network care isn't covered unless it's an emergency.

- **POS (Point of Service Plan):** This one's a bit of a hybrid. Like an HMO, you need a PCP referral to see a specialist, but you can also go outside the network like a PPO, though at a higher cost.

Understanding Premiums, Deductibles, Co-pays, and Co-insurance

- **Premium:** The monthly fee you pay for your insurance. Consider it like a subscription fee.

- **Deductible:** The amount you pay for healthcare services before your insurance kicks in.

- **Co-pay:** A fixed amount you pay for a healthcare service, like a ticket price, while the insurance covers the rest.

- **Co-insurance:** This is a bit like splitting a bill. It's the percentage of the healthcare costs you pay after meeting your deductible.

Why is Eligibility Verification Important?

Eligibility verification is like checking the weather before heading out. It ensures that the patient's insurance is active and covers the services they need. This step is crucial to avoid billing surprises down the road – both for the healthcare provider and the patient.

In conclusion, understanding these health insurance concepts is like having a map of the maze. It gives you the knowledge to navigate the complexities of medical insurance eligibility verification confidently. With this map in hand, we're ready to delve deeper into the maze in the upcoming sections.

1.2 Types of Health Insurance Plans

As we continue our journey through the maze of medical insurance, it's time to explore the different paths one can take – the various types of health insurance plans. Each type has its unique features, benefits, and limitations, much like choosing a path in a sprawling garden, with each leading to different experiences.

HMO: Health Maintenance Organization

- **Characteristics:** With an HMO, you're part of a network with a primary care physician (PCP) who is your main healthcare guide.

- **Referrals:** Need referrals from your PCP to see specialists.

- **Cost:** Generally lower premiums and co-pays, but less flexibility in choosing providers.

- **Ideal for:** Those who prefer a straightforward, coordinated approach to healthcare and don't mind the limitations on provider choice.

PPO: Preferred Provider Organization

- **Characteristics:** PPOs offer more freedom to choose your healthcare providers.

- **Referrals:** No need for referrals to see specialists.

- **Cost:** Usually higher premiums and co-pays but more choice and flexibility.

- **Ideal for:** Individuals wanting more control over their healthcare choices and willing to pay a bit more for that flexibility.

EPO: Exclusive Provider Organization

- **Characteristics:** EPO plans combine elements of HMO and PPO. You can choose any provider within a network without a referral.

- **Cost:** Generally, lower costs than PPOs but with less flexibility than PPOs and more than HMOs.

- **Out-of-Network Care:** Not covered unless it's an emergency.

- **Ideal for:** Those who value some choice but don't mind the limitation of staying within a network.

POS: Point of Service Plan

- **Characteristics:** A mix between HMO and PPO. You have a PCP, but you can also go out-of-network.

- **Referrals:** Required for specialists, similar to HMOs.

- **Cost:** Generally higher out-of-pocket costs if you go out-of-network.

- **Ideal for:** People who are comfortable with a PCP coordinating their care but also want the freedom to go outside the network when needed.

High-Deductible Health Plans (HDHPs) with Health Savings Accounts (HSAs)

- **Characteristics:** Higher deductible plans that can be paired with an HSA, allowing you to save money tax-free for medical expenses.

- **Cost:** Lower premiums, but higher out-of-pocket costs until the deductible is met.

- **Ideal for:** Those with fewer medical expenses who can benefit from the savings aspect.

Medicare and Medicaid

- **Medicare:** A federal program primarily for people aged 65 and older or with certain disabilities.

- **Medicaid:** State and federal program for individuals and families with lower incomes.

Understanding Your Plan

Knowing your health insurance plan is like having the right key for a treasure chest. It helps in unlocking the right healthcare services without unexpected financial surprises. Each plan type offers different paths in your healthcare journey, and choosing the right one depends on your health needs, financial situation, and preferences in healthcare management.

As we continue our exploration, the importance of this understanding becomes even clearer, especially when it comes to eligibility verification – a crucial step in ensuring that the healthcare services align seamlessly with the coverage provided by these diverse insurance plans.

1.3 The Importance of Eligibility Verification in Healthcare

Diving deeper into the healthcare insurance maze, we arrive at a crucial checkpoint – eligibility verification. It's like the guardrail of the healthcare system, ensuring that every step forward is on solid ground. Let's explore why this process is so pivotal in healthcare.

Ensuring Coverage and Avoiding Denials

Imagine a patient receiving healthcare services only to find out later that their insurance doesn't cover those services. It's like reaching the end of a maze and finding a locked door. Eligibility verification prevents this by confirming in advance that the patient's insurance plan covers the specific services they need. This step is crucial in avoiding claim denials and ensuring smooth billing and payment processes.

Facilitating Financial Planning

For both healthcare providers and patients, understanding the financial aspect is as essential as a compass in navigation. Eligibility verification helps patients understand their financial responsibilities upfront, be it copays, deductibles, or out-of-pocket maximums. For healthcare providers, it's about ensuring that the services provided will be compensated, thereby maintaining a steady financial flow.

Improving Patient Satisfaction and Trust

There's nothing more disheartening for patients than unexpected medical bills. By verifying eligibility at the outset, healthcare providers can foster transparency and trust. This clarity enhances patient satisfaction, as patients feel more secure and informed about their healthcare journey.

Reducing Administrative Burdens

Eligibility verification streamlines the administrative process. It reduces the time and resources spent on managing billing errors and claim resubmissions. Efficient verification processes mean less administrative burden and more focus on patient care.

Enhancing Healthcare Efficiency

Proper verification leads to fewer delays and disruptions. It's like oiling the gears of the healthcare machine – everything runs more smoothly when everyone is aware of and prepared for the financial aspects of healthcare services.

Compliance with Regulations

In the world of healthcare, numerous regulations govern billing and insurance claims. Eligibility verification helps in adhering to these regulations by ensuring that claims are accurate and compliant, thus avoiding legal and financial repercussions.

In Conclusion

Eligibility verification is more than just a procedural step; it’s a fundamental aspect of healthcare that upholds the integrity and efficiency of the entire system. As we navigate further into the realms of medical insurance eligibility verification, the significance of this process becomes increasingly apparent – it's the cornerstone upon which reliable and effective healthcare services are built.

1.4 Exercise: 10 MCQs with Answers at the End

1. **What is the primary purpose of eligibility verification in healthcare?**

A. To provide entertainment to patients

B. To ensure insurance coverage aligns with provided services

C. To increase the time spent on administrative tasks

D. To complicate the billing process

2. **Eligibility verification helps in avoiding:**

A. Patient satisfaction

B. Claim denials

C. Efficient healthcare delivery

D. Use of modern technology

3. **What aspect of patient care is enhanced by upfront eligibility verification?**

A. Confusion about services

B. Financial transparency and trust

C. Unnecessary treatments

D. Patient entertainment

4. **Eligibility verification is crucial for understanding:**

A. The latest fashion trends

B. A patient's financial responsibility for services

C. Only the patient's medical history

D. The interior design of the clinic

5. **Which of the following is a benefit of eligibility verification for healthcare providers?**

A. Increased claim denials

B. Improved patient-physician relationships

C. Reduced administrative burdens

D. Higher operational costs

6. **Efficient eligibility verification processes primarily lead to:**

A. More time spent on administrative tasks

B. Less focus on patient care

C. Fewer delays and disruptions in healthcare service delivery

D. Increased patient anxiety

7. **In terms of regulations, eligibility verification helps in:**

A. Ignoring compliance requirements

B. Adhering to healthcare billing and insurance regulations

C. Decreasing the accuracy of claims

D. Complicating legal matters

8. **One reason eligibility verification is important is that it:**

A. Decreases the efficiency of healthcare services

B. Increases the financial risk for patients

C. Ensures compensation for healthcare services

D. Limits the use of digital technology in healthcare

9. **The process of eligibility verification affects:**

A. Only the healthcare providers

B. Both healthcare providers and patients

C. Only the insurance companies

D. None of the above

10. **A key outcome of proper eligibility verification is:**

A. Increased financial ambiguity

B. Lower patient satisfaction

C. Enhanced transparency in financial matters

D. More frequent claim denials

Answers

1. **B. To ensure insurance coverage aligns with provided services**
2. **B. Claim denials**
3. **B. Financial transparency and trust**
4. **B. A patient's financial responsibility for services**
5. **C. Reduced administrative burdens**
6. **C. Fewer delays and disruptions in healthcare service delivery**
7. **B. Adhering to healthcare billing and insurance regulations**
8. **C. Ensures compensation for healthcare services**
9. **B. Both healthcare providers and patients**
10. **C. Enhanced transparency in financial matters**

Chapter 2: The Verification Process

2.1 Steps in the Insurance Verification Process

Embarking on the next stage of our journey in the realm of medical insurance eligibility verification, let's navigate the critical steps in the insurance verification process. Think of it as a treasure hunt, where each step brings us closer to the prize: a seamless, efficient healthcare experience for both providers and patients.

Step 1: Collection of Patient Information

- **Initial Stage:** The journey begins with the collection of patient information. This includes basic details like name, date of birth, and insurance ID.

- **Accuracy is Key:** Ensuring the accuracy of this information is crucial – think of it as setting the right coordinates for a successful voyage.

Step 2: Verification of Insurance Coverage

- **Contacting the Insurer:** Next, contact the patient's insurance company, either online or via phone, to verify coverage.

- **Checking Details:** Confirm details like coverage start and end dates, benefits, co-pay amounts, deductibles, and out-of-pocket maximums.

Step 3: Determining Patient's Financial Responsibility

- **Informed Estimates:** Based on the verified information, determine the patient's financial responsibility. This includes any co-pays, co-insurance, or deductibles that the patient needs to be aware of.

- **Clear Communication:** Communicating this information to patients upfront can prevent surprises and build trust.

Step 4: Identifying Authorization Requirements

- **Pre-Authorization:** Some treatments or services may require pre-authorization from the insurance company.

- **Timely Requests:** Identifying and obtaining these authorizations in advance ensures that the services provided are covered.

Step 5: Documentation

- **Record Keeping:** Document all the verified information and any communication with the insurance company. This step is the safety net, ensuring that if there's ever a question or dispute, you have the necessary information at hand.

- **Confidentiality:** Maintain confidentiality and compliance with healthcare regulations, such as HIPAA.

Step 6: Regular Updates and Re-verification

- **Stay Updated:** Insurance details can change, so it's important to re-verify coverage regularly, especially for ongoing treatments.

- **Proactive Approach:** This step is like regularly checking your map to ensure you're still on the right path.

In conclusion, the insurance verification process is a detailed and crucial pathway in the healthcare journey. Each step requires careful attention to ensure accuracy, compliance, and clear communication. By meticulously following these steps, healthcare providers can minimize billing errors, reduce claim denials, and enhance the overall patient experience. It's a process that, when executed well, leads to a treasure trove of patient satisfaction and efficient healthcare delivery.

2.2 Best Practices for Efficient Verification

As we continue to navigate the intricate process of insurance verification, it's essential to adopt best practices that streamline the journey, making it more efficient and reliable. These best practices are like the guiding stars in the night sky, leading to a smoother verification process.

Start with Accurate Patient Information

- **Precision at the Outset:** Ensure that patient information is accurately collected at the first point of contact. This includes double-checking names, dates of birth, and insurance details.

- **Use of Technology:** Utilize electronic health records (EHRs) and other software to capture and store patient information, reducing the chances of errors.

Leverage Technology for Verification

- **Automated Verification Tools:** Employ automated insurance verification tools to speed up the process. These tools can quickly check patient coverage details, saving time and reducing manual errors.

- **Integration with EHRs:** Integrate verification tools with electronic health records for a streamlined process.

Stay Informed About Insurance Policies

- **Continuous Education:** Keep the team updated on changes in insurance policies and healthcare regulations. This knowledge is crucial for accurate verification.

- **Regular Training:** Conduct regular training sessions for staff on the latest trends and updates in health insurance.

Clear Communication with Patients

- **Upfront Information:** Clearly communicate with patients about their insurance coverage and financial responsibilities. This transparency helps in building trust and preventing misunderstandings.

- **Patient Education:** Educate patients about how their insurance works, especially regarding co-pays, deductibles, and out-of-pocket costs.

Efficient Record-Keeping and Documentation

- **Meticulous Records:** Maintain detailed records of all verifications and communications with insurance providers. This documentation is vital for resolving any disputes or clarifications.

- **Confidentiality and Compliance:** Ensure that all records are kept confidential and in compliance with HIPAA and other relevant regulations.

Develop a Systematic Follow-Up Process

- **Regular Updates:** Implement a system for regular re-verification of insurance, especially for patients with ongoing treatment plans.

- **Proactive Approach:** Anticipate and resolve potential issues before they become problems, such as expiring authorizations or changes in coverage.

Foster Strong Relationships with Insurance Companies

- **Collaborative Approach:** Develop and maintain positive relationships with insurance providers. Good rapport can facilitate smoother interactions and quicker resolutions.

Continuous Process Improvement

- **Feedback Mechanisms:** Encourage feedback from staff and patients to identify areas for improvement.

- **Quality Checks:** Regularly review the verification process for any inefficiencies or recurring issues, and adjust procedures accordingly.

Adopting these best practices in insurance verification is like fine-tuning a well-oiled machine. It ensures that each step of the process runs smoothly, leading to increased accuracy, patient satisfaction, and operational efficiency. With these guidelines in place, the journey through the maze of insurance verification becomes much more navigable, benefitting both healthcare providers and patients.

2.3 Common Challenges in Eligibility Verification

Navigating the twists and turns of insurance eligibility verification, like any intricate process, comes with its own set of challenges. These hurdles can often slow down or complicate the journey. Understanding these common obstacles is crucial for developing strategies to effectively overcome them.

Complexity of Insurance Policies

- **Variability:** Insurance policies can be as varied and complex as a labyrinth. They often have different coverage rules, exclusions, and benefits, making verification a meticulous task.

- **Frequent Changes:** Insurance plans and benefits can change regularly, adding another layer of complexity to staying current.

Patient Information Inaccuracies

- **Data Entry Errors:** Simple mistakes in patient data entry, such as misspelled names or incorrect policy numbers, can lead to significant issues in eligibility verification.

- **Outdated Information:** Patients may not always provide the most current insurance information, leading to discrepancies during verification.

Lack of Patient Understanding

- **Insurance Complexity:** Many patients have a limited understanding of their own insurance policies, which can lead to confusion and incorrect assumptions about coverage.

- **Communication Gaps:** Miscommunication about insurance benefits and patient responsibilities can lead to misunderstandings and dissatisfaction.

Time Constraints and Workload

- **High Volume:** High patient volumes can strain the verification process, especially in busy healthcare settings.

- **Time-Intensive Process:** The need for detailed verification for each patient can be time-consuming, impacting workflow efficiency.

Technological Limitations

- **Outdated Systems:** Not all healthcare facilities have access to the latest technology for automated verification, relying instead on manual processes that are more prone to error.

- **Integration Issues:** Challenges in integrating verification tools with existing electronic health records or billing systems can complicate the process.

Insurance Company Delays and Errors

- **Response Times:** Delays in responses from insurance companies can hold up the verification process.

- **Incorrect Information:** Errors or outdated information from insurance providers can lead to incorrect eligibility determinations.

Regulatory Compliance Issues

- **Keeping Up with Regulations:** Navigating the myriad of healthcare regulations and ensuring compliance adds another layer of complexity to the verification process.

- **Privacy Concerns:** Maintaining patient privacy and adhering to regulations like HIPAA during the verification process is paramount and challenging.

In conclusion, while the path of insurance eligibility verification is fraught with challenges, understanding and acknowledging these issues is the first step in addressing them. By recognizing these common obstacles, healthcare providers can develop more efficient strategies and systems to streamline the verification process, ensuring accuracy, compliance, and a smoother journey for both providers and patients.

2.4 Exercise: 10 MCQs with Answers at the End

1. **What is a major challenge in eligibility verification due to the nature of insurance policies?**

A. Their simplicity and consistency

B. Variability and frequent changes

C. Lack of any detailed guidelines

D. The colorfulness of insurance brochures

2. **A common issue with patient information that affects eligibility verification is:**

A. Perfect accuracy

B. Data entry errors

C. Overly detailed information

D. Excessive brevity in patient responses

3. **Lack of patient understanding in insurance matters often leads to:**

A. High levels of patient satisfaction

B. Miscommunication about coverage

C. Faster verification processes

D. More accurate self-diagnoses

4. **Which factor significantly strains the eligibility verification process in busy healthcare settings?**

A. Low patient volumes

B. High patient volumes

C. Excessive leisure time among staff

D. Over-automation of processes

5. **What technological challenge can impede efficient eligibility verification?**

A. Over-reliance on manual processes

B. Too much reliance on artificial intelligence

C. Use of highly advanced software only

D. Excessive internet speeds

6. **Delays and errors from which party can disrupt the verification process?**

A. Insurance companies

B. Food delivery services

C. Internet service providers

D. Postal services

7. **A major regulatory concern in eligibility verification is:**

A. Adhering to fashion trends

B. Ensuring compliance with healthcare regulations

C. Following sports rules

D. Keeping up with movie releases

8. **How does high volume of patients affect the verification process?**

A. Makes it less time-consuming

B. Reduces workload

C. Can lead to time constraints and increased workload

D. Enhances the enjoyment of the process

9. **Outdated technology in healthcare facilities can lead to:**

A. Improved accuracy in verification

B. Increased reliance on efficient manual processes

C. Challenges in performing eligibility verification

D. Faster processing times

10. **One of the key challenges in dealing with insurance companies during verification is:**

A. Their prompt and error-free responses

B. Delays in responses and potential for incorrect information

C. Their entertaining communication style

D. The frequency of their social media updates

Answers

1. **B. Variability and frequent changes**
2. **B. Data entry errors**
3. **B. Miscommunication about coverage**
4. **B. High patient volumes**
5. **A. Over-reliance on manual processes**
6. **A. Insurance companies**

7. **B. Ensuring compliance with healthcare regulations**

8. **C. Can lead to time constraints and increased workload**

9. **C. Challenges in performing eligibility verification**

10. **B. Delays in responses and potential for incorrect information**

Chapter 3: Navigating Insurance Terminologies

3.1 Key Insurance Terms and Definitions

Embarking on the third chapter of our journey, we enter the dense forest of insurance terminologies. Understanding these terms is akin to having a translator in a foreign land; it makes navigation through the complex world of insurance more comprehensible and less daunting.

Premium

- **Definition:** The premium is the amount you pay for your health insurance every month. Think of it as a subscription fee to keep your insurance active.

- **Impact on Coverage:** It's important to pay this regularly to maintain coverage and avoid policy lapses.

Deductible

- **Definition:** This is the amount you pay out of pocket for healthcare services before your insurance starts to pay. It's like the initial investment in a game before the rewards kick in.

- **Considerations:** High-deductible plans usually have lower premiums, but they mean more out-of-pocket costs upfront.

Co-Payment (Co-pay)

- **Definition:** A co-pay is a fixed amount you pay for a specific service or medication. It's similar to a fixed ticket price for a specific ride in an amusement park.

- **Usage:** Common in HMO plans, co-pays are typically paid at the time of the service.

Co-Insurance

- **Definition:** Co-insurance is your share of the costs of a healthcare service, usually calculated as a percentage. It's like splitting the bill at a restaurant after a deductible is met.

- **Example:** If you have 20% co-insurance, you pay 20% of the cost of a healthcare service, and your insurance covers the rest.

Out-of-Pocket Maximum

- **Definition:** This is the most you have to pay for covered services in a plan year. After reaching this limit, your insurance pays 100% for covered services.

- **Safety Net:** It acts as a financial safety net, preventing excessive spending in a year, particularly in case of major health issues.

Network

- **Definition:** A network refers to the group of doctors, hospitals, and other healthcare providers that your insurance plan has contracted with to provide services at a negotiated rate.

- **Types:** In-network (part of the plan's network) and out-of-network (not part of the plan's network) providers can have different costs associated.

Pre-Authorization

- **Definition:** This is a decision by your health insurer that a healthcare service, treatment plan, prescription drug, or durable medical equipment is medically necessary.

- **Prior Approval:** Some services require pre-authorization from your insurance company before they can be provided.

Explanation of Benefits (EOB)

- **Definition:** An EOB is a statement from your insurance company after you receive a healthcare service, explaining what was covered and what you may owe.

- **Clarification Tool:** It's not a bill but a helpful tool to understand the insurance claim and any charges you may be responsible for.

In conclusion, navigating these key insurance terms is essential for both healthcare providers and patients. It ensures a better understanding of how health insurance works, clarifies financial responsibilities, and aids in making informed decisions about healthcare services. With this knowledge, we can confidently continue our exploration into the more intricate aspects of medical insurance eligibility verification.

3.2 Decoding Insurance Benefits and Coverage

As we delve deeper into the forest of insurance jargon, it's time to decode the often enigmatic realm of insurance benefits and coverage. Understanding this is like deciphering a complex code that unlocks the true value and limitations of a health insurance plan.

Understanding Insurance Benefits

- **Scope of Coverage:** Insurance benefits outline what types of medical services, treatments, or drugs are covered under a plan. It's the list of what's included in your insurance package.

- **Preventive Services:** Many plans cover preventive services like vaccinations, screenings, and annual check-ups, often at no cost to the patient.

- **Specialized Care:** Benefits also detail coverage for specialized care, such as maternity services, mental health treatment, and emergency services.

Determining Coverage Limits

- **Annual and Lifetime Limits:** Some plans set limits on how much they will pay for your health services over a year or over your lifetime. Knowing these limits is crucial to avoid unexpected expenses.

- **Benefit Caps:** Certain services may have benefit caps, which limit the amount the insurance will pay for specific treatments.

Decoding Coverage Exclusions

- **Non-Covered Services:** Every insurance plan has exclusions, which are services not covered. Understanding what's excluded is as important as knowing what's covered.

- **Elective Procedures:** Common exclusions often include elective or cosmetic procedures and alternative therapies.

Understanding Network Restrictions

- **In-Network vs. Out-of-Network:** Insurance plans often have a network of providers. Using in-network providers usually costs you less, whereas out-of-network services can lead to higher out-of-pocket expenses.

- **Referral Requirements:** Some plans, especially HMOs, may require a referral from your primary care physician to see a specialist.

Checking Prescription Drug Coverage

- **Formulary:** Most plans have a formulary, a list of covered prescription drugs. It's vital to check whether your medications are on this list and understand the co-pays or co-insurance associated with them.

Evaluating Additional Benefits

- **Wellness Programs:** Some insurance plans offer additional benefits like discounts on gym memberships, weight loss programs, or wellness activities.

- **Telehealth Services:** With the rise of digital health, many plans now include telehealth services, allowing virtual consultations and treatments.

Navigating Policy Changes

- **Annual Updates:** Insurance plans can change annually, so it's important to review your benefits each year during the enrollment period.

- **Staying Informed:** Keeping abreast of policy changes helps in maximizing benefits and avoiding surprises.

In conclusion, decoding insurance benefits and coverage is a critical step in understanding the full scope of what your health insurance offers. It empowers patients to make informed healthcare choices and enables healthcare providers to advise patients accurately on coverage and financial responsibilities. With this key knowledge, we are better equipped to navigate the complex healthcare landscape.

3.3 Understanding Exclusions and Limitations

In the complex tapestry of health insurance, exclusions and limitations are like the knots that can trip you up if you're not careful. This chapter is about understanding these critical aspects of insurance plans, which dictate what is not covered or only partially covered.

Identifying Exclusions in Insurance Policies

- **Definition:** Exclusions are specific conditions or services that an insurance policy does not cover. They are the 'not covered' list.

- **Common Exclusions:** These often include cosmetic surgeries, experimental treatments, and non-emergency care when traveling outside the country.

Understanding Coverage Limitations

- **Definition:** Limitations are restrictions on the extent or amount of coverage for certain services or treatments within an insurance policy.

- **Examples:** Limitations can come in the form of caps on the number of visits (like physical therapy sessions), duration limits (such as short-term rehabilitation services), or dollar limits on certain services.

Navigating Lifetime and Annual Limits

- **Lifetime Limits:** Some insurance plans set a maximum amount they will pay for your healthcare over the lifetime of the policy.

- **Annual Limits:** These are caps on the amount an insurance plan will pay in a given policy year. Post-ACA, most essential health benefits cannot have annual or lifetime dollar limits.

Handling Benefit Caps

- **Implications:** Benefit caps can affect how much insurance will pay for specific treatments, often leaving the patient to cover the rest.

- **Strategies:** Understanding these caps helps in financial planning, especially for treatments that involve ongoing care.

Dealing with Pre-Existing Conditions

- **Pre-ACA Challenges:** Prior to the Affordable Care Act (ACA), pre-existing conditions often led to coverage exclusions or higher rates.

- **Post-ACA Landscape:** The ACA prohibits denial of coverage due to pre-existing conditions, but it's crucial to understand how these conditions are handled in your plan.

Evaluating Excluded Medications

- **Formulary Lists:** Each insurance plan has a formulary that lists which medications are covered. Medications not on this list are typically excluded.

- **Generic vs. Brand-Name:** Insurance might cover a generic version of a medication, but not the brand-name version, or vice versa.

Policy Changes and Updates

- **Staying Informed:** Insurance policies can change annually, so it's important to review your policy regularly to stay informed about any new exclusions or limitations.

Conclusion

Understanding exclusions and limitations is critical in managing expectations regarding healthcare coverage. It helps in making informed decisions about healthcare choices and financial planning. By being aware of these aspects, patients can avoid surprises related to uncovered services, and healthcare providers can better guide their patients in navigating their healthcare journey.

3.4 Exercise: 10 MCQs with Answers at the End

1. **Insurance exclusions refer to:**

A. Services fully covered by the insurance.

B. The range of services partially covered.

C. Specific conditions or services not covered by the policy.

D. The premium amount of the insurance.

2. **Which of the following is often an exclusion in health insurance policies?**

A. Emergency treatments.

B. Cosmetic surgeries.

C. Primary care visits.

D. Inpatient hospital services.

3. **Coverage limitations in insurance policies typically:**

A. Increase the premium.

B. Extend coverage to additional services.

C. Restrict the extent or amount of coverage for certain services.

D. Apply only to external healthcare providers.

4. **What are lifetime limits in health insurance policies?**

A. Limits on the number of insurance policies one can hold.

B. Caps on the total amount the policy will pay over the policyholder's lifetime.

C. Restrictions on the age at which one can purchase insurance.

D. The maximum duration for which a policy can be held.

5. **Annual limits in health insurance policies are:**

A. Caps on the amount an insurance plan will pay in a given policy year.

B. The annual premium amount payable.

C. Limits on the number of hospital visits per year.

D. Restrictions on the number of claims in a year.

6. **Benefit caps in health insurance typically affect:**

A. The insurance company's profits.

B. The design of the insurance card.

C. How much insurance will pay for specific treatments.

D. The availability of healthcare providers.

7. **Prior to the Affordable Care Act (ACA), insurance policies:**

A. Were required to cover pre-existing conditions.

B. Often excluded coverage for pre-existing conditions.

C. Provided additional benefits for pre-existing conditions.

D. Were not available to individuals with pre-existing conditions.

8. **Post-ACA, insurance policies:**

A. Can exclude pre-existing conditions.

B. Cannot deny coverage due to pre-existing conditions.

C. Have increased premiums for pre-existing conditions.

D. Provide limited coverage for pre-existing conditions.

9. **A medication not listed in an insurance plan's formulary is typically:**

A. Covered with higher co-pays.

B. Excluded from coverage.

C. Covered under special circumstances.

D. Available without any cost.

10. **Why is it important to regularly review your health insurance policy?**

A. To check for any increase in premium.

B. To ensure understanding of new exclusions or limitations.

C. To change the insurance provider.

D. To decrease the coverage amount.

Answers

1. **C. Specific conditions or services not covered by the policy.**

2. **B. Cosmetic surgeries.**

3. **C. Restrict the extent or amount of coverage for certain services.**

4. **B. Caps on the total amount the policy will pay over the policyholder's lifetime.**

5. **A. Caps on the amount an insurance plan will pay in a given policy year.**

6. **C. How much insurance will pay for specific treatments.**

7. **B. Often excluded coverage for pre-existing conditions.**

8. **B. Cannot deny coverage due to pre-existing conditions.**

9. **B. Excluded from coverage.**

10. **B. To ensure understanding of new exclusions or limitations.**

Chapter 4: The Role of Technology in Verification

4.1 Electronic Verification Systems

As we venture further into the intricate world of medical insurance eligibility verification, the role of technology, particularly electronic verification systems, emerges as a game-changer. These systems are akin to having a high-tech compass in an explorer's toolkit, making the journey through the complex terrain of insurance verification smoother and more efficient.

What are Electronic Verification Systems?

- **Definition:** Electronic Verification Systems are technology solutions designed to automate the process of verifying patient insurance coverage.

- **Functionality:** They connect healthcare providers directly to insurance payers, offering real-time access to insurance eligibility data.

Benefits of Electronic Verification Systems

- **Increased Efficiency:** Automation speeds up the verification process, significantly reducing the time required to confirm patient coverage.

- **Accuracy:** These systems minimize human error, ensuring more accurate verification results.

- **Reduced Administrative Burden:** By automating routine tasks, staff can focus on more complex aspects of patient care and billing.

Features of Electronic Verification Systems

- **Real-Time Data Access:** Access to up-to-date patient eligibility and benefits information.

- **Integration with EHRs:** Many systems integrate seamlessly with existing Electronic Health Records (EHRs), centralizing patient data and streamlining workflow.

- **Customizable Alerts and Notifications:** Alerts for important information like lapses in coverage or changes in patient eligibility.

Implementation Considerations

- **Training and Adoption:** Proper training for staff to use these systems effectively.

- **Cost and ROI Analysis:** Evaluating the cost of implementation against the potential return on investment, considering factors like reduced claim denials and improved cash flow.

- **Data Security and Compliance:** Ensuring the system meets all regulatory compliance requirements, especially regarding patient data privacy (HIPAA compliance).

Choosing the Right Electronic Verification System

- **Needs Assessment:** Determining the specific needs of your healthcare practice.

- **Vendor Evaluation:** Researching and comparing different vendors to find a system that aligns with your workflow and budget.

- **Scalability and Support:** Considering the system's scalability for future growth and the level of customer support provided by the vendor.

The Future of Electronic Verification

- **Advanced Technologies:** Incorporation of advanced technologies like AI and machine learning for more predictive and intelligent verification processes.

- **Interoperability:** Enhanced interoperability between different healthcare systems for more cohesive data exchange and verification processes.

In conclusion, electronic verification systems are transforming the landscape of insurance verification in healthcare. By embracing these technological solutions, healthcare providers can achieve greater accuracy, efficiency, and patient satisfaction in the verification process. It’s a step towards a more technologically integrated and streamlined future in healthcare management.

4.2 The Impact of Digitalization on Insurance Verification

The digital revolution has transformed numerous industries, and healthcare insurance verification is no exception. In this chapter, we explore how the digitalization wave has reshaped the insurance verification process, akin to a technological renaissance that has brought about efficiency, speed, and accuracy.

Enhanced Efficiency and Speed

- **Automation:** Digital tools have automated the labor-intensive and time-consuming tasks of insurance verification, much like shifting from manual labor to automated machinery in manufacturing.

- **Rapid Verification:** With digital systems, what used to take hours or days can now be accomplished in minutes. This speed is crucial in fast-paced healthcare environments where timely patient care is paramount.

Increased Accuracy and Reduced Errors

- **Error Reduction:** Digitalization minimizes human errors that can occur in manual verification processes. Automated systems are less prone to overlooking critical details or misinterpreting information.

- **Consistency:** Digital tools provide consistent and standardized verification processes, ensuring uniformity in handling insurance verifications across various patients and services.

Improved Patient Experience

- **Quicker Service:** The quick turnaround in verification processes leads to shorter wait times and more efficient patient intake processes.

- **Transparency:** Digital tools can provide patients with clear, real-time information about their insurance coverage and financial responsibilities, enhancing transparency and trust.

Data Analytics and Insights

- **Trend Analysis:** Digitalization allows for the collection and analysis of vast amounts of data, enabling healthcare providers to identify trends, such as common reasons for claim denials or patient coverage issues.

- **Informed Decision-Making:** With data analytics, healthcare facilities can make informed decisions about their operational strategies and patient care processes.

Cost-Effectiveness

- **Reduced Operational Costs:** By streamlining the verification process, digital tools help in reducing administrative costs associated with manual verification.

- **Revenue Cycle Improvement:** Accurate and efficient verification processes contribute to a more robust and reliable revenue cycle, reducing the likelihood of claim denials and delayed payments.

Challenges in the Digital Transition

- **Adoption Barriers:** Some healthcare providers may face challenges in adopting new technologies, whether due to cost, resistance to change, or lack of technical expertise.

- **Training and Adaptation:** Ensuring that staff are adequately trained and comfortable with new digital systems is crucial for successful implementation.

Conclusion

The impact of digitalization on insurance verification is profound and multi-faceted. It has revolutionized the way healthcare providers interact with insurance companies and manage patient information, leading to a more streamlined, efficient, and patient-friendly process. As technology continues to evolve, its role in further simplifying and enhancing insurance verification processes will undoubtedly expand, paving the way for more innovations in healthcare management.

4.3 Future Trends in Insurance Technology

In the dynamic landscape of healthcare, insurance technology is not just keeping pace but is often at the forefront of innovation. As we peer into the crystal ball of insurance tech, several future trends emerge, promising to further revolutionize the way eligibility verification and other insurance-related processes are handled.

Artificial Intelligence and Machine Learning

- **Predictive Analytics:** AI and machine learning are set to transform insurance verification by predicting coverage issues and suggesting solutions before they arise.

- **Automated Decision-Making:** These technologies can enable more sophisticated decision-making processes, analyzing vast datasets to optimize verification and billing practices.

Blockchain Technology

- **Enhanced Security:** Blockchain could provide unparalleled security for storing and sharing patient insurance data, ensuring integrity and confidentiality.

- **Smart Contracts:** The use of blockchain-based smart contracts could automate many aspects of insurance verification and claims processing, reducing time and eliminating errors.

Internet of Things (IoT)

- **Connected Healthcare Devices:** IoT devices could automatically update patient records and insurance information, ensuring real-time data accuracy.

- **Remote Patient Monitoring:** IoT devices can facilitate remote monitoring, which can be directly linked to insurance providers for seamless claim processing based on real-time patient data.

Telemedicine and Digital Health Services

- **Expansion of Coverage:** As telemedicine continues to grow, insurance providers will likely expand coverage for digital health services, necessitating updates in verification processes.

- **Integration with Verification Systems:** Seamless integration of telehealth platforms with insurance verification systems could streamline the process for remote healthcare services.

Mobile Health (mHealth) Applications

- **Patient Empowerment:** mHealth apps can empower patients by providing easy access to their insurance information, eligibility status, and benefit details.

- **Real-Time Verification:** These apps could allow for real-time insurance verification and updates, making healthcare access more efficient for patients on the go.

Voice Technology and Chatbots

- **Automated Customer Service:** Voice-activated technology and chatbots could handle routine insurance verification inquiries, freeing up human resources for more complex tasks.

- **Enhanced Patient Interaction:** These technologies can provide a more interactive and user-friendly way for patients to understand their insurance coverage and obligations.

Personalized Insurance Plans

- **Customization Based on Data:** Big data analytics could lead to more personalized insurance plans tailored to individual health needs and preferences, affecting the way eligibility is verified and managed.

- **Dynamic Coverage Options:** Insurance plans could become more dynamic, adjusting coverage based on real-time health data and lifestyle changes.

Conclusion

The future of insurance technology in healthcare is bright and brimming with potential. These advancements promise not only enhanced efficiency and accuracy in insurance verification processes but also a more patient-centric approach to healthcare. As these technologies evolve, they will inevitably shape a new era in healthcare administration, where innovation leads to better patient care and streamlined operations.

4.4 Exercise: 10 MCQs with Answers at the End

1. **What technology is predicted to play a significant role in future insurance verification processes?**

A. Artificial Intelligence (AI) and Machine Learning

B. Fax machines

C. Typewriters

D. Rotary phones

2. **Blockchain technology in insurance verification could enhance:**

A. Paper-based record-keeping

B. Security and confidentiality of data

C. Manual data entry processes

D. Postal mail efficiency

3. **The Internet of Things (IoT) in healthcare could contribute to:**

A. Decreasing the use of technology in medicine

B. Automatic updating of patient records and insurance information

C. Reducing internet connectivity

D. Eliminating the need for doctors

4. **How might telemedicine impact insurance verification?**

A. By eliminating the need for insurance

B. By reducing the use of technology in healthcare

C. By expanding coverage for digital health services

D. By increasing in-person doctor visits

5. **Mobile Health (mHealth) applications can:**

A. Make insurance verification more difficult

B. Provide patients easy access to their insurance information

C. Discourage the use of smartphones

D. Increase paper-based healthcare processes

6. **Voice technology and chatbots in healthcare can:**

A. Only play music for patients

B. Handle routine insurance verification inquiries

C. Reduce internet usage

D. Complicate patient interaction

7. **Future personalized insurance plans may be influenced by:**

A. Patients' fashion choices

B. Big data analytics

C. Preference for outdated technology

D. Dislike of modern medicine

8. **What is a potential benefit of AI and machine learning in insurance verification?**

A. Decreasing data accuracy

B. Predicting coverage issues before they arise

C. Slowing down the verification process

D. Reducing the use of computers

9. **Blockchain-based smart contracts in insurance could:**

A. Increase the need for manual verification

B. Automate aspects of insurance verification and claims processing

C. Eliminate digital data storage

D. Decrease data security

10. **Which technology could provide real-time insurance verification updates for mobile users?**

A. Mobile Health (mHealth) applications

B. Pagers

C. Public payphones

D. Radio broadcasts

Answers

1. **A. Artificial Intelligence (AI) and Machine Learning**

2. **B. Security and confidentiality of data**

3. **B. Automatic updating of patient records and insurance information**

4. **C. By expanding coverage for digital health services**

5. **B. Provide patients easy access to their insurance information**

6. **B. Handle routine insurance verification inquiries**

7. **B. Big data analytics**

8. **B. Predicting coverage issues before they arise**

9. **B. Automate aspects of insurance verification and claims processing**

10. **A. Mobile Health (mHealth) applications**

Chapter 5: Communication with Insurance Providers

5.1 Effective Communication Strategies

In the realm of medical insurance verification, effective communication with insurance providers is akin to navigating a dialogue in a complex dance. It requires tact, clarity, and strategic understanding. This chapter delves into the art of effective communication strategies that can streamline interactions and facilitate a smoother verification process.

Establishing Clear Channels of Communication

- **Direct Lines:** Establish direct lines of communication, such as dedicated phone numbers or email addresses, for queries and clarifications.

- **Point of Contact:** Identify specific contacts or departments within insurance companies for different types of inquiries.

Developing a Professional Rapport

- **Relationship Building:** Foster professional relationships with representatives from insurance companies. Like any good relationship, this can lead to better cooperation and understanding.

- **Consistent Interactions:** Regular and predictable communication helps in building trust and efficiency.

Utilizing Technology for Communication

- **Electronic Communication:** Leverage secure email, portals, and messaging systems for exchanging information. This can speed up responses and provide a written record.

- **Automated Updates:** Utilize automated systems for receiving updates from insurance providers, such as changes in policies or coverage.

Effective Query Resolution

- **Specific Inquiries:** Be specific and clear in your queries to avoid back-and-forth communication. Clarity is key in obtaining the right information.

- **Follow-up Procedures:** Establish a follow-up protocol for unresolved queries or when awaiting a response. Timely follow-ups can prevent delays in patient care and billing.

Training and Education

- **Staff Training:** Ensure staff are well-trained in insurance terminologies, policies, and procedures. Knowledge empowers them to communicate effectively and confidently.

- **Regular Updates:** Keep the team updated on changes in the insurance landscape, which can impact communication strategies and requirements.

Documentation and Record-Keeping

- **Accurate Records:** Maintain detailed records of all communications with insurance providers. This documentation is invaluable for resolving disputes and clarifying agreements.

- **Privacy Compliance:** Ensure all communication adheres to privacy laws and regulations, such as HIPAA.

Effective Listening and Responsiveness

- **Active Listening:** Practice active listening during interactions. Understanding the perspective of the insurance provider can aid in resolving issues more effectively.

- **Prompt Responses:** Respond promptly to queries from insurance providers. This not only builds a positive rapport but can also expedite the verification process.

Conclusion

Effective communication with insurance providers is a critical component of the insurance verification process. It enhances the efficiency, clarity, and reliability of interactions, leading to smoother operations and better outcomes. By mastering these communication strategies, healthcare providers can navigate the complex insurance landscape with greater ease and effectiveness.

5.2 Handling Denials and Appeals

Navigating through the intricacies of insurance denials and appeals is an essential skill in the healthcare industry. This process can be compared to solving a complex puzzle where each piece must be meticulously placed for a successful outcome. Let's explore the strategies for effectively handling denials and managing the appeals process.

Understanding the Reasons for Denials

- **Initial Step:** The first step in handling a denial is to understand why it occurred. Common reasons include lack of coverage, non-adherence to policy guidelines, or errors in claim submission.

- **Detailed Review:** Carefully review the denial notice, which should provide specific reasons for the rejection.

Effective Communication Post-Denial

- **Contacting the Insurance Provider:** Reach out to the insurance company for a more detailed explanation if the denial reasons are unclear. Clear communication can often clarify misunderstandings or provide additional insight.

- **Internal Review:** Discuss the denial with relevant healthcare team members to gather additional insights or identify any internal errors.

Preparation for the Appeal Process

- **Gathering Documentation:** Collect all necessary documentation, including medical records, prior authorization, and any relevant correspondence.

- **Understanding Appeal Procedures:** Each insurance provider has specific procedures for filing an appeal. Familiarize yourself with these guidelines to ensure compliance.

Writing the Appeal Letter

- **Clear and Concise:** Write a clear and concise appeal letter. State the reasons for the appeal and include evidence to support your case.

- **Supporting Evidence:** Attach all relevant documentation to strengthen the appeal. This may include medical notes, test results, or a letter of medical necessity from the healthcare provider.

Monitoring the Appeal Process

- **Tracking:** Keep a detailed record of the appeal submission, including dates and correspondence.

- **Follow-up:** Regular follow-up is key. Establish a timeline for follow-up calls or emails to check on the status of the appeal.

Learning from Denials

- **Review and Analysis:** Analyze denied claims to identify any patterns or common issues. This can provide valuable insights for reducing future denials.

- **Staff Training:** Use denial data as a learning tool to train staff on common pitfalls and best practices for claim submission.

Developing a Proactive Approach

- **Prevention Strategies:** Develop strategies to minimize denials, such as double-checking for common errors or ensuring that all necessary pre-authorization requirements are met.

- **Staying Informed:** Keep abreast of changes in insurance policies and guidelines that might affect claim submissions and approvals.

Conclusion

Effectively handling denials and appeals is a critical component of revenue cycle management in healthcare. By understanding the reasons behind denials, preparing thoroughly for appeals, and learning from past experiences, healthcare providers can enhance their efficiency and success rate in navigating these challenges. This proactive and informed approach not only improves financial outcomes but also ensures that patients receive the care they need without undue administrative burdens.

5.3 Building Relationships with Insurance Companies

Navigating the complex world of healthcare insurance isn't just about understanding policies and procedures; it's also about building and maintaining positive relationships with insurance companies. Just as a gardener nurtures plants to ensure their best growth, healthcare providers must cultivate relationships with insurers for mutual benefit and smoother operations.

Establishing a Foundation of Trust and Communication

- **Open Dialogue:** Foster open lines of communication. Regular interaction can build trust and facilitate easier resolution of issues.

- **Understanding Perspectives:** Recognize the challenges and constraints that insurance companies face. This understanding can lead to more empathetic and productive interactions.

Networking and Regular Interactions

- **Attend Industry Events:** Engage with insurance representatives at healthcare conferences and seminars. These interactions outside of the office setting can strengthen professional relationships.

- **Regular Meetings:** Schedule periodic meetings or calls with insurance company representatives to discuss common issues, updates, or changes in policies.

Collaborative Problem-Solving

- **Joint Efforts:** Work together on common challenges, such as reducing claim denials or streamlining the verification process. Collaboration can lead to innovative solutions.

- **Feedback Exchange:** Provide constructive feedback and be open to receiving it as well. This two-way communication can improve processes on both ends.

Training and Education

- **Informed Staff:** Ensure that your staff are well-trained in the specifics of different insurance plans and company policies. Knowledgeable interactions reflect positively on your organization.

- **Insurance Education:** Invite insurance representatives to conduct training sessions for your staff. This can provide valuable insights directly from the source.

Responsiveness and Reliability

- **Prompt Responses:** Be prompt in responding to requests or inquiries from insurance companies. Timeliness is a key component of a good working relationship.

- **Accurate Information:** Ensure that all information provided to insurance companies is accurate and complete. Reliability builds trust.

Developing Personal Connections

- **Personal Rapport:** Beyond professional interactions, develop a personal rapport with insurance representatives. Understanding each other on a personal level can facilitate smoother professional interactions.

- **Appreciation and Recognition:** Acknowledge the efforts and assistance provided by insurance representatives. A little appreciation can go a long way in maintaining positive relationships.

Adapting to Changes

- **Stay Informed:** Keep abreast of changes in the insurance industry and adapt your practices accordingly. Being proactive in adjusting to changes shows your commitment to a seamless partnership.

- **Flexibility:** Be flexible in your interactions and negotiations with insurance companies. Flexibility can often lead to more mutually beneficial outcomes.

Conclusion

Building and maintaining strong relationships with insurance companies is an invaluable aspect of efficient healthcare management. These relationships can lead to better communication, fewer misunderstandings, and more effective problem-solving. Like any good relationship, it requires effort, understanding, and commitment, but the payoff is a smoother, more effective insurance verification process and better overall healthcare delivery.

5.4 Exercise: 10 MCQs with Answers at the End

1. **Effective communication with insurance companies is essential for:**

A. Increasing entertainment in the workplace.

B. Building trust and facilitating issue resolution.

C. Reducing internet usage.

D. Enhancing office decor.

2. **Attending industry events and seminars helps in building relationships with insurance companies by:**

A. Providing a venue for leisure activities.

B. Engaging with insurance representatives outside the office.

C. Reducing the need for communication.

D. Increasing sales of unrelated products.

3. **Collaborative problem-solving with insurance companies can lead to:**

A. More complex issues.

B. Innovative solutions to common challenges.

C. Decreased efficiency.

D. Ignoring important issues.

4. **The purpose of inviting insurance representatives for staff training is to:**

A. Promote the insurance company's products.

B. Provide insights directly from the source.

C. Increase the workload of staff.

D. Focus on non-healthcare related topics.

5. **What is a key component of maintaining a good working relationship with insurance companies?**

A. Avoiding communication.

B. Providing inaccurate information.

C. Being prompt in responses.

D. Reducing the number of meetings.

6. **Personal rapport with insurance representatives can:**

A. Complicate professional interactions.

B. Facilitate smoother professional interactions.

C. Lead to unnecessary gossip.

D. Decrease the importance of formal communication.

7. **In building relationships with insurance companies, flexibility is important because it:**

A. Increases bureaucratic procedures.

B. Often leads to more mutually beneficial outcomes.

C. Reduces the need for understanding policies.

D. Encourages ignoring rules.

8. **Feedback exchange with insurance companies is vital for:**

A. Creating a competitive environment.

B. Improving processes and communication.

C. Reducing collaboration.

D. Focusing only on the negatives.

9. **A proactive approach in adapting to changes in the insurance industry shows:**

A. A lack of commitment to healthcare delivery.

B. Commitment to a seamless partnership.

C. Unwillingness to learn.

D. Disregard for industry standards.

10. **Why is accurate information provision to insurance companies crucial?**

A. It has no real impact.

B. To maintain a sense of mystery.

C. For building trust and reliability.

D. To increase paperwork.

Answers

1. **B. Building trust and facilitating issue resolution.**

2. **B. Engaging with insurance representatives outside the office.**

3. **B. Innovative solutions to common challenges.**

4. **B. Provide insights directly from the source.**

5. **C. Being prompt in responses.**

6. **B. Facilitate smoother professional interactions.**

7. **B. Often leads to more mutually beneficial outcomes.**

8. **B. Improving processes and communication.**

9. **B. Commitment to a seamless partnership.**

10. **C. For building trust and reliability.**

Chapter 6: Legal and Regulatory Aspects

6.1 Compliance with Healthcare Laws

In the realm of healthcare, navigating the legal and regulatory aspects is akin to sailing through a sea governed by stringent laws. Compliance with healthcare regulations is not just a legal obligation but a critical aspect of maintaining trust and integrity in healthcare practices. In this chapter, we delve into the essentials of compliance with healthcare laws in the context of insurance verification.

Understanding Healthcare Regulations

- **HIPAA:** The Health Insurance Portability and Accountability Act (HIPAA) is a cornerstone of healthcare privacy laws. It regulates the use and disclosure of Protected Health Information (PHI).

- **Affordable Care Act (ACA):** ACA regulations impact various aspects of insurance coverage, including eligibility criteria and coverage mandates.

Importance of Compliance

- **Patient Trust:** Compliance ensures the confidentiality and security of patient data, which is fundamental in maintaining patient trust.

- **Avoiding Legal Repercussions:** Non-compliance can lead to legal penalties, including fines and sanctions, which can be detrimental to healthcare providers both financially and reputationally.

Training and Education

- **Staff Training:** Regular training sessions for staff on HIPAA and other healthcare laws are crucial. This ensures that everyone is aware of their responsibilities regarding patient data and insurance processing.

- **Updates on Changes:** Healthcare laws are subject to change. Keeping abreast of these changes and updating policies and procedures accordingly is essential.

Implementing Compliance Protocols

- **Privacy Policies:** Establishing robust privacy policies that govern how patient information is handled and shared.

- **Regular Audits:** Conducting regular audits to ensure compliance with healthcare laws and identifying areas for improvement.

Record Keeping and Documentation

- **Accurate Records:** Maintaining accurate and detailed records is a key aspect of compliance. This includes documentation of insurance verifications, communications with insurance companies, and patient consent forms.

- **Access Controls:** Implementing strict access controls to ensure that only authorized personnel have access to sensitive patient information.

Dealing with Breaches

- **Response Plan:** Have a clear plan in place for responding to any breaches of patient data. This includes steps for notification, containment, and remediation.

- **Reporting:** Understanding the reporting requirements in case of a breach and ensuring timely compliance with these requirements.

Conclusion

Compliance with healthcare laws is a fundamental aspect of insurance verification and healthcare delivery. It's about more than just adhering to rules; it's about upholding ethical standards and ensuring the safety and privacy of patient information. By prioritizing legal and regulatory compliance, healthcare providers not only protect themselves from legal risks but also fortify the trust and confidence of their patients.

6.2 Understanding HIPAA in Insurance Verification

The Health Insurance Portability and Accountability Act (HIPAA) is a critical framework in the healthcare industry, particularly in the realm of insurance verification. Understanding and adhering to HIPAA regulations is like navigating a river with strong currents – it requires precision and a deep understanding of the guidelines to ensure a smooth and compliant journey.

HIPAA Overview

- **Purpose:** HIPAA was enacted to protect the privacy and security of individuals' medical information, known as Protected Health Information (PHI).

- **Scope:** It applies to all healthcare providers, insurance companies, and healthcare clearinghouses that handle PHI.

HIPAA in the Context of Insurance Verification

- **Privacy Rule:** The Privacy Rule restricts the use and disclosure of PHI without patient consent, which is paramount during the insurance verification process.

- **Minimum Necessary Standard:** When verifying insurance, only the minimum necessary information should be used or disclosed to accomplish the intended purpose.

Patient Rights Under HIPAA

- **Access to Records:** Patients have the right to access their medical records, including information used for insurance verification.

- **Amendments to Records:** Patients can request corrections to their PHI if inaccuracies are identified.

Compliance in Insurance Verification

- **Training Staff:** Ensure that all staff involved in the insurance verification process are trained in HIPAA compliance.

- **Securing PHI:** Implement security measures to protect PHI, including secure electronic transmission and storage of data.

- **Patient Consent:** Obtain necessary authorizations or consents from patients before using or disclosing their PHI for insurance verification.

Handling PHI

- **Disclosure Guidelines:** Be cautious about what information is disclosed during the insurance verification process. Ensure that any disclosure aligns with HIPAA requirements.

- **Verification Requests:** When requesting verification from insurers, ensure that the request aligns with HIPAA's minimum necessary standard.

Dealing with HIPAA Violations

- **Violation Identification:** Regularly monitor and audit insurance verification processes to identify potential HIPAA violations.

- **Immediate Action:** In the event of a violation, take immediate action to rectify the situation and prevent future occurrences.

- **Reporting Requirements:** Understand the reporting requirements and timelines in the case of a breach of PHI.

Conclusion

Understanding and complying with HIPAA in the insurance verification process is not just a legal obligation but also a crucial aspect of maintaining patient trust and safeguarding their sensitive information. It requires ongoing vigilance, regular training, and a commitment to uphold the highest standards of privacy and security. By adhering to HIPAA guidelines, healthcare providers can ensure that their insurance verification processes are not only efficient but also respectful of patients' rights and privacy.

6.3 The Impact of Healthcare Reforms on Insurance Eligibility

Healthcare reforms, particularly significant legislative changes like the Affordable Care Act (ACA), have had a profound impact on insurance eligibility and the landscape of healthcare in the United States. Understanding these reforms is akin to charting a course through new waters, requiring a clear grasp of how these changes influence insurance eligibility processes.

Expansion of Coverage Under ACA

- **Mandatory Coverage:** One of the key aspects of the ACA was the individual mandate, which required most Americans to have health insurance or face a penalty. This expanded the pool of insured individuals.

- **Medicaid Expansion:** The ACA allowed for the expansion of Medicaid eligibility to cover more low-income individuals and families, significantly increasing the number of people eligible for insurance.

Changes in Insurance Policy Requirements

- **Pre-Existing Conditions:** The ACA prohibited insurance companies from denying coverage or charging higher rates based on pre-existing conditions. This broadened eligibility for many who were previously denied insurance.

- **Essential Health Benefits:** The ACA established a set of essential health benefits that all insurance plans must cover, impacting the scope of coverage available to policyholders.

Implications for Insurance Verification

- **Broader Eligibility Checks:** With more individuals insured and changes in policy requirements, insurance verification processes must be more comprehensive and thorough.

- **Updated Verification Protocols:** Healthcare providers have had to update their insurance verification protocols to align with the changes brought about by healthcare reforms.

Impact on Insurance Marketplaces

- **Establishment of Exchanges:** The ACA led to the creation of health insurance marketplaces or exchanges, offering a variety of plans. This requires healthcare providers to be familiar with a broader range of insurance options during the verification process.

Influence on Patient Demographics

- **Diverse Patient Population:** The expansion of insurance coverage has led to a more diverse patient population accessing healthcare services, necessitating adaptations in the insurance verification process to cater to different needs.

Continued Adaptation to Reforms

- **Ongoing Changes:** Healthcare reforms are subject to political and legislative changes. Healthcare providers must stay informed about current regulations and adapt their insurance verification processes accordingly.

Conclusion

The impact of healthcare reforms on insurance eligibility has been significant, requiring healthcare providers to adapt and update their verification processes. These reforms have broadened access to healthcare, necessitating a more comprehensive understanding of various insurance plans and eligibility criteria. Staying informed and adaptable is crucial for healthcare providers to navigate these changes effectively and ensure that patients receive the coverage they are entitled to under the reformed healthcare landscape.

6.4 Exercise: 10 MCQs with Answers at the End

1. **The Affordable Care Act (ACA) expanded healthcare coverage by:**

A. Reducing the number of insured individuals.

B. Introducing the individual mandate.

C. Eliminating Medicaid.

D. Decreasing the essential health benefits.

2. **Under the ACA, insurance companies are prohibited from:**

A. Providing online services.

B. Denying coverage based on pre-existing conditions.

C. Offering multiple plan options.

D. Conducting healthcare research.

3. **One impact of healthcare reforms on insurance verification is:**

A. A decrease in the need for thorough checks.

B. Narrower eligibility checks.

C. More comprehensive and thorough eligibility checks.

D. Elimination of insurance verification.

4. **The ACA's Medicaid expansion primarily aimed to:**

A. Reduce coverage for low-income individuals.

B. Increase coverage for more low-income individuals and families.

C. Limit healthcare services to specific groups.

D. Privatize healthcare services.

5. **Essential Health Benefits under the ACA are:**

A. Optional for insurance plans to cover.

B. A set of benefits that all insurance plans must cover.

C. Only available in certain states.

D. Limited to emergency services.

6. **Health insurance marketplaces or exchanges were established to:**

A. Decrease the variety of insurance plans available.

B. Offer a variety of insurance plans.

C. Increase healthcare costs.

D. Limit patient choice in healthcare.

7. **Since the implementation of the ACA, insurance verification processes must be:**

A. Less comprehensive.

B. More focused on elderly patients.

C. More comprehensive and thorough.

D. Exclusively automated.

8. **The individual mandate in the ACA refers to:**

A. A requirement for most Americans to have health insurance.

B. A mandate for individuals to pay higher premiums.

C. A suggestion to consider health insurance.

D. The choice of opting out of all health insurance.

9. **Adapting to healthcare reforms in insurance verification involves:**

A. Ignoring changes in regulations.

B. Staying informed about current regulations.

C. Reducing the scope of verification.

D. Focusing solely on private insurance plans.

10. **The expansion of Medicaid eligibility affects insurance verification by:**

A. Limiting the number of people who can be Insured.

B. Increasing the complexity of eligibility checks.

C. Simplifying insurance policies.

D. Decreasing the diversity of the patient population.

Answers

1. **B. Introducing the individual mandate.**

2. **B. Denying coverage based on pre-existing conditions.**

3. **C. More comprehensive and thorough eligibility checks.**

4. **B. Increase coverage for more low-income individuals and families.**

5. **B. A set of benefits that all insurance plans must cover.**

6. **B. Offer a variety of insurance plans.**

7. **C. More comprehensive and thorough.**

8. **A. A requirement for most Americans to have health insurance.**

9. **B. Staying informed about current regulations.**

10. **B. Increasing the complexity of eligibility checks.**

Chapter 7: Verification in Different Healthcare Settings

7.1 Hospitals vs. Private Practices

The process of insurance verification, while fundamentally similar, can vary significantly between different healthcare settings, particularly when comparing hospitals and private practices. These variations are like the difference between navigating a large ocean liner and a small sailboat – both navigate the same waters, but their approaches and challenges can be quite different.

Insurance Verification in Hospitals

- **Complexity and Volume:** Hospitals typically deal with a higher volume of patients and more complex cases, making the insurance verification process more intricate.

- **Diverse Insurance Plans:** Due to the variety of services offered, hospitals encounter a broader range of insurance plans and coverage types.

- **Specialized Departments:** Larger hospitals often have dedicated departments for insurance verification, with specialized staff for different types of insurance or treatments.

- **Technology and Integration:** Hospitals are more likely to use advanced technology for verification, which may be integrated with other hospital information systems for comprehensive patient management.

Insurance Verification in Private Practices

- **Personalized Approach:** Private practices often have a more direct relationship with their patients, allowing for a more personalized approach to insurance verification.

- **Limited Staff Resources:** Smaller practices may have fewer staff members who handle multiple roles, including insurance verification.

- **Simpler Insurance Interactions:** Private practices typically deal with a smaller variety of insurance plans, which can simplify the verification process.

- **Focus on Specific Services:** The scope of services in private practices is usually more focused, which can streamline the verification process for specific insurance requirements related to those services.

Common Challenges and Solutions

- **Resource Allocation:** Hospitals need to allocate sufficient resources to handle the volume and complexity, whereas private practices may need to prioritize efficiency due to limited staff.

- **Technology Utilization:** Both settings can benefit from using electronic verification tools, though the scale and integration level might differ.

- **Training and Knowledge:** Continuous training in insurance policies and verification procedures is crucial in both settings to ensure accuracy and compliance.

- **Patient Communication:** Clear communication with patients about their insurance coverage and financial responsibilities is essential, irrespective of the healthcare setting.

Conclusion

Insurance verification in hospitals and private practices has its unique set of challenges and requirements. Understanding these differences is key to developing effective verification strategies tailored to each setting. While hospitals may navigate the complexities of a vast array of insurance issues with more resources, private practices often steer through these challenges with a more personal touch and focused approach. In both cases, the goal remains the same: to ensure accurate and efficient insurance verification for optimal patient care and smooth administrative processes.

7.2 Specialty-Specific Verification Challenges

In the diverse landscape of healthcare, different medical specialties encounter unique challenges in insurance verification. Just as a cardiologist and a dermatologist face different clinical challenges, their insurance verification processes also present distinct hurdles. Let's explore these specialty-specific challenges and how they impact the insurance verification process.

Cardiology

- **High-Cost Procedures:** Cardiology often involves expensive procedures and tests, making accurate insurance verification crucial to ensure coverage.

- **Pre-Authorization Requirements:** Many cardiac procedures require pre-authorization due to their high costs and complexity.

Oncology

- **Long-Term Treatment Plans:** Cancer treatment typically involves long-term plans, requiring ongoing verification to ensure continuous coverage.

- **Specialty Drugs:** Oncology often uses expensive specialty drugs that may have specific insurance requirements or limited coverage.

Orthopedics

- **Elective Surgeries:** Many orthopedic procedures are elective, which may or may not be covered by insurance.

- **Durable Medical Equipment:** Orthopedic treatments often require the use of durable medical equipment (DME), which has its own set of insurance verification challenges.

Mental Health

- **Varied Coverage Levels:** Mental health services can have varying levels of coverage, with some plans offering limited sessions or higher copays.

- **Stigma and Privacy Concerns:** There may be additional sensitivity around the verification process due to the stigma associated with mental health treatment.

Pediatrics

- **Family Insurance Policies:** Verifying coverage for children can be complex, especially under family insurance plans with different coverage details for dependents.

- **Vaccinations and Regular Check-ups:** Regular pediatric services like vaccinations and wellness check-ups often have specific coverage rules.

Dermatology

- **Cosmetic vs. Medical Treatments:** Distinguishing between cosmetic procedures (typically not covered) and medical treatments is a key aspect of verification in dermatology.

- **Topical Medications:** Insurance coverage for dermatological prescriptions can vary greatly, requiring careful verification.

Challenges Across Specialties

- **Staying Informed:** Specialists must stay informed about the specific insurance requirements and changes related to their field.

- **Patient Communication:** Clear communication with patients about the coverage of specialized procedures and potential out-of-pocket costs is crucial.

- **Efficient Processes:** Developing efficient verification processes to handle the specific demands of each specialty.

Conclusion

Specialty-specific challenges in insurance verification require tailored approaches to ensure effective and accurate coverage confirmation. Each specialty faces its own set of hurdles, from high-cost procedures in cardiology to the nuances of coverage in mental health services. Understanding these unique challenges is essential for healthcare providers in each specialty to navigate the insurance verification process successfully and ensure optimal patient care.

7.3 Verification in Dental and Vision Care

In the world of healthcare, dental and vision care present unique challenges in the insurance verification process. Unlike general healthcare, which often deals with a broad range of medical issues, dental and vision care are specialized fields with specific insurance considerations. Understanding these nuances is crucial for accurate and effective insurance verification in these areas.

Dental Insurance Verification

- **Separate Insurance Plans:** Often, dental coverage is separate from general health insurance plans, requiring specific verification processes.

- **Annual Maximums:** Dental plans typically have annual maximums, which limit the amount the insurer will pay within a given year.

- **Variability in Coverage:** Coverage for dental procedures can vary significantly, with preventative care often covered at a higher percentage than major procedures like crowns or bridges.

- **Waiting Periods:** Some dental insurance plans have waiting periods for certain procedures, which must be verified to avoid unexpected patient charges.

Challenges in Dental Verification

- **Understanding Plan Limitations:** Verifying specific details like annual maximums, co-pays, and covered percentages for various procedures.

- **Frequency of Services:** Regular treatments like cleanings and check-ups require ongoing verification throughout the year.

Vision Insurance Verification

- **Specialized Coverage:** Vision insurance often covers specific services like eye exams, glasses, or contact lenses, separate from other medical care.

- **Limited Benefits:** Many vision plans offer benefits that are limited to certain frequencies, such as one eye exam per year or glasses every two years.

- **Combination with Medical Insurance:** In cases of medical eye issues (not routine care), vision care might be covered under the patient's general medical insurance, necessitating dual verification.

Challenges in Vision Verification

- **Clarifying Coverage:** Differentiating between routine vision care and medical eye care, as the insurance coverage can differ.

- **Product-Specific Limitations:** Verifying coverage for specific products, such as types of lenses or frames, which may have distinct limitations or allowances.

Best Practices for Verification in Dental and Vision Care

- **Detailed Inquiry:** Given the specificity of coverage, detailed inquiries into the extent and limitations of the coverage are essential.

- **Regular Updates:** Since benefits and allowances reset annually or biannually, regularly updating verification processes is crucial.

- **Clear Patient Communication:** Informing patients clearly about their coverage, out-of-pocket costs, and any potential limitations or waiting periods.

Conclusion

Verification in dental and vision care requires a specialized approach due to the unique nature of these insurance plans. By understanding the intricacies of dental and vision insurance, healthcare providers in these fields can ensure accurate verification, thereby enhancing patient satisfaction and minimizing billing issues. This specialized approach is key to navigating the specific challenges presented by dental and vision insurance verification.

7.4 Exercise: 10 MCQs with Answers at the End

1. **Dental insurance plans typically:**

A. Have no annual maximums.

B. Include coverage for all procedures.

C. Have annual maximums limiting the amount paid per year.

D. Cover all procedures at 100%.

2. **In dental insurance verification, a significant aspect to check is:**

A. The patient's favorite color.

B. Annual maximums and coverage for specific procedures.

C. The brand of dental equipment used.

D. The dentist's years of experience.

3. **Vision insurance often covers:**

A. All medical treatments.

B. Only dental procedures.

C. Specific services like eye exams and glasses.

D. Every healthcare need.

4. **A unique challenge in vision insurance verification is:**

   A. Determining coverage for routine versus medical eye care.

   B. Verifying the color of the patient's eyes.

   C. Checking the weather on the day of the appointment.

   D. Deciding the brand of eye drops.

5. **Waiting periods in dental insurance refer to:**

   A. Time spent in the waiting room.

   B. Periods before certain procedures are covered.

   C. Delays in appointment scheduling.

   D. Time taken for a dental procedure.

6. **For vision care, it is important to differentiate between:**

   A. Different brands of contact lenses.

   B. Routine vision care and medical eye care.

C. The patient's vision dreams.

D. Types of vision tests.

7. **In dental care, preventative procedures are usually covered:**

A. At a lower percentage than major procedures.

B. Not at all.

C. At a higher percentage than major procedures.

D. Only if the patient insists.

8. **Benefits and allowances in vision insurance typically:**

A. Change daily.

B. Have no set frequency or limitation.

C. Reset annually or biannually.

D. Increase with each visit.

9. **A best practice for dental and vision insurance verification is:**

A. Assuming coverage is the same as medical insurance.

B. Detailed inquiries into coverage extent and limitations.

C. Ignoring annual maximums.

D. Focusing solely on the cost of procedures.

10. **Clear patient communication in dental and vision care is important to inform patients about:**

A. Unrelated medical facts.

B. Coverage, out-of-pocket costs, and potential limitations.

C. The history of dentistry and optometry.

D. The interior design of the clinic.

Answers

1. **C. Have annual maximums limiting the amount paid per year.**

2. **B. Annual maximums and coverage for specific procedures.**

3. **C. Specific services like eye exams and glasses.**

4. **A. Determining coverage for routine versus medical eye care.**

5. **B. Periods before certain procedures are covered.**

6. **B. Routine vision care and medical eye care.**

7. **C. At a higher percentage than major procedures.**

8. **C. Reset annually or biannually.**

9. **B. Detailed inquiries into coverage extent and limitations.**

10. **B. Coverage, out-of-pocket costs, and potential limitations.**

Chapter 8: Managing Patient Expectations and Experience

8.1 Educating Patients About Their Insurance

In the healthcare journey, managing patient expectations and experience is pivotal, akin to a navigator guiding a ship through unfamiliar waters. A key aspect of this is educating patients about their insurance, which empowers them to make informed decisions and sets realistic expectations about their care and associated costs.

Importance of Patient Education on Insurance

- **Enhancing Understanding:** Many patients have limited knowledge about the specifics of their insurance coverage. Educating them can demystify the complexities of insurance benefits, limitations, and their financial responsibilities.

- **Preventing Billing Surprises:** Knowledge about insurance coverage helps prevent unexpected medical bills, enhancing patient satisfaction and trust.

Strategies for Educating Patients

- **Simplified Explanations:** Use simple, non-technical language to explain insurance terms and benefits. Complex jargon can be more confusing than helpful.

- **Personalized Discussions:** Tailor the discussion to the specific services the patient will receive, explaining how their insurance will cover these services.

- **Visual Aids:** Utilize brochures, charts, or digital tools to visually demonstrate insurance coverage and costs.

Incorporating Insurance Education in Patient Interactions

- **At Registration:** Start the conversation about insurance during the patient registration process.

- **During Appointments:** Providers can reinforce insurance information during medical appointments, especially when discussing treatment plans.

- **Follow-up Communication:** Provide written summaries or follow-up communications that reiterate key insurance information.

Addressing Common Patient Queries

- **Deductibles and Co-pays:** Explain how deductibles, co-pays, and co-insurance work, and how they affect out-of-pocket costs.

- **Coverage Limits and Exclusions:** Discuss common coverage limits and exclusions that might be relevant to the patient's care.

- **Pre-Authorization Requirements:** Inform patients about the need for pre-authorization for certain procedures and how it impacts their treatment timeline.

Leveraging Technology for Education

- **Patient Portals:** Use patient portals to provide access to insurance information, coverage details, and educational materials.

- **Mobile Apps:** Encourage the use of insurance provider apps where patients can easily check their coverage, benefits, and claim status.

Conclusion

Educating patients about their insurance is a critical step in managing expectations and enhancing the overall patient experience. It involves clear communication, personalized discussions, and effective use of educational tools and technology. By equipping patients with a better understanding of their insurance coverage, healthcare providers can foster a more transparent, trusting, and satisfying healthcare journey.

8.2 Strategies to Enhance Patient Satisfaction

Patient satisfaction is a cornerstone of quality healthcare service. It's akin to a favorable review in a customer-oriented business, reflecting the healthcare provider's commitment to exceptional care and service. Let's explore strategies that can enhance patient satisfaction, particularly in the context of managing their expectations and experiences with insurance and healthcare services.

Effective Communication

- **Clear and Compassionate Dialogue:** Consistently communicate in a clear, compassionate manner. Patients value understanding and empathy as much as they value the technical competence of their healthcare providers.

- **Active Listening:** Pay close attention to patients' concerns and questions, demonstrating that their views and experiences are valued and understood.

Transparency in Costs and Procedures

- **Upfront Information:** Provide patients with detailed information about the costs of treatment, insurance coverage, and potential out-of-pocket expenses. Transparency helps in building trust and avoiding unpleasant surprises.

- **Explain Medical Procedures:** Clearly explain medical procedures, what they entail, and their importance. Patients who understand their medical journey feel more comfortable and involved.

Personalized Patient Care

- **Individualized Attention:** Treat each patient as an individual with unique needs and preferences. Personalized care significantly enhances patient satisfaction.

- **Patient-Centered Approach:** Focus on delivering care that is respectful of and responsive to individual patient preferences, needs, and values.

Efficient Service Delivery

- **Minimize Wait Times:** Strive to minimize wait times, both in scheduling appointments and in waiting rooms. Efficient service delivery is a key contributor to patient satisfaction.

- **Streamlined Administrative Processes:** Ensure that administrative processes, such as registration and billing, are as seamless and patient-friendly as possible.

Utilizing Technology

- **Digital Tools for Engagement:** Employ digital tools like patient portals, apps, and telemedicine services to enhance patient engagement and convenience.

- **Online Resources:** Provide access to online resources for health education, appointment scheduling, and health monitoring.

Feedback Mechanisms

- **Patient Surveys and Feedback:** Regularly solicit feedback from patients through surveys or comment forms. Patient feedback is invaluable for understanding and addressing areas that need improvement.

- **Responsive to Feedback:** Show that the healthcare facility is responsive to feedback by implementing changes where necessary and communicating these changes back to patients.

Continuous Staff Training

- **Professional Development:** Regularly train staff in customer service, communication skills, and empathy. The attitude and behavior of every staff member impact patient satisfaction.

- **Awareness of Best Practices:** Keep staff updated on best practices in patient care and satisfaction.

Creating a Comfortable Environment

- **Welcoming Atmosphere:** Ensure that the healthcare environment is clean, comfortable, and welcoming. The physical environment plays a significant role in patient perceptions.

- **Supportive Services:** Offer supportive services, such as patient navigators or counselors, to help patients through their healthcare journey.

Conclusion

Enhancing patient satisfaction is a multifaceted endeavor that involves effective communication, transparency, personalized care, efficiency, and the use of modern technology. By adopting these strategies, healthcare providers can create a more positive, reassuring, and satisfying experience for patients, leading to better healthcare outcomes and stronger patient-provider relationships.

8.3 Handling Patient Queries on Coverage and Benefits

Effectively addressing patient queries about insurance coverage and benefits is a critical aspect of healthcare service. It's akin to being a knowledgeable guide in a complex terrain, helping patients navigate through the often confusing landscape of insurance policies. Here are strategies for efficiently handling patient questions regarding their coverage and benefits.

Establish a Knowledgeable Frontline

- **Trained Staff:** Ensure that the staff responsible for patient interaction, especially at the front desk and billing departments, are well-trained in insurance policies and can competently address basic insurance queries.

- **Resource Availability:** Keep insurance policy summaries and FAQs readily available for staff reference.

Effective Communication Techniques

- **Simplifying Information:** Use simple, non-technical language to explain complex insurance terms and coverage details.

- **Active Listening:** Listen carefully to understand the specific concerns or queries of the patient, providing targeted and relevant information.

Utilizing Educational Materials

- **Brochures and Leaflets:** Provide easy-to-understand brochures or leaflets that outline common insurance terms, coverage basics, and how to understand benefits.

- **Digital Resources:** Offer access to online resources where patients can learn about their insurance coverage and benefits.

Personalized Responses

- **Individual Assessment:** Assess each patient's situation individually and provide information specific to their coverage plan and healthcare needs.

- **Clarification of Benefits:** Clearly explain what is covered under their plan, including any exclusions or limitations that are particularly relevant to their treatment or services.

Streamlining Inquiry Responses

- **Centralized Information Hub:** Create a centralized database or repository of information on various insurance plans and benefits for quick reference.

- **Template Responses:** Develop template responses for frequently asked questions to ensure consistency and efficiency in providing information.

Collaboration with Insurance Companies

- **Direct Contact:** In cases of complex queries, facilitate direct contact between the patient and their insurance provider, or offer to contact the insurer on the patient's behalf.

- **Regular Updates:** Keep abreast of changes and updates in insurance policies to provide the most current information to patients.

Managing Expectations

- **Transparent Communication:** Be upfront about the limitations of the information provided, emphasizing that final coverage decisions rest with the insurance company.

- **Guidance on Next Steps:** Advise patients on the next steps if their coverage is unclear or if they need to take further action with their insurance provider.

Conclusion

Handling patient queries about insurance coverage and benefits is about more than just providing information; it's about enhancing patient understanding, trust, and satisfaction. By employing these strategies, healthcare providers can assist patients in making informed decisions about their care and manage expectations regarding insurance coverage and financial responsibilities.

8.4 Exercise: 10 MCQs with Answers at the End

1. **Effective handling of patient queries about insurance is crucial for:**

A. Increasing patient confusion.

B. Enhancing patient understanding and satisfaction.

C. Lengthening appointment times.

D. Selling insurance policies.

2. **What should staff do when faced with complex insurance queries?**

A. Guess the answers.

B. Refer to detailed insurance policy summaries and FAQs.

C. Ignore the questions.

D. Offer unrelated advice.

3. **When explaining insurance terms and coverage to patients, it's important to:**

A. Use complex medical jargon.

B. Simplify the information using non-technical language.

C. Speak in a foreign language.

D. Provide information only in written form.

4. **Providing brochures and leaflets about insurance helps in:**

A. Complicating the insurance understanding.

B. Marketing new insurance products.

C. Outlining common insurance terms and coverage basics.

D. Increasing paper waste in the clinic.

5. **A personalized response to an insurance query should include:**

A. General information irrelevant to the patient's specific situation.

B. Details specific to the patient's coverage plan and healthcare needs.

C. Promotional material for different insurance plans.

D. Only the benefits of the most expensive procedures.

6. **Why is it beneficial to have a centralized database of insurance information?**

A. To increase the workload on staff.

B. For quick reference and efficient response to inquiries.

C. To collect data for marketing purposes.

D. To avoid answering patient questions.

7. **How should healthcare providers handle complex insurance queries that they cannot answer?**

A. Make up an answer.

B. Facilitate direct contact between the patient and their insurance provider.

C. Tell the patient it's not their concern.

D. Change the subject.

8. **Managing patient expectations in insurance inquiries involves:**

A. Promising coverage for all treatments.

B. Being upfront about the limitations of the information provided.

C. Guaranteeing that the insurance will pay for everything.

D. Offering discounts on treatments.

9. **Template responses for frequently asked insurance questions ensure:**

A. Each patient gets a unique answer.

B. Inconsistency in information.

C. Consistency and efficiency in providing information.

D. Patients become more confused.

10. **What is a key aspect of streamlining inquiry responses?**

A. Providing the same generic answer to all questions.

B. Developing a centralized information hub.

C. Avoiding detailed explanations.

D. Encouraging patients to not ask questions.

Answers

1. **B. Enhancing patient understanding and satisfaction.**
2. **B. Refer to detailed insurance policy summaries and FAQs.**
3. **B. Simplify the information using non-technical language.**
4. **C. Outlining common insurance terms and coverage basics.**
5. **B. Details specific to the patient's coverage plan and healthcare needs.**
6. **B. For quick reference and efficient response to inquiries.**
7. **B. Facilitate direct contact between the patient and their insurance provider.**
8. **B. Being upfront about the limitations of the information provided.**
9. **C. Consistency and efficiency in providing information.**
10. **B. Developing a centralized information hub.**

Chapter 9: Revenue Cycle Management and Insurance Verification

9.1 Role of Verification in Revenue Cycle

In the intricate ecosystem of healthcare finance, the role of insurance verification in revenue cycle management is both pivotal and multifaceted. It's akin to laying the foundation for a building – essential for the stability and success of the entire structure. Let's delve into how insurance verification interplays with and influences the revenue cycle in healthcare.

Understanding the Revenue Cycle

- **Definition:** The revenue cycle in healthcare encompasses all the financial processes related to patient care, from initial appointment scheduling to final payment collection.

- **Critical Phases:** It includes patient registration, insurance verification, charge capture, claim submission, payment posting, and accounts receivable management.

Impact of Insurance Verification on the Revenue Cycle

- **Upfront Verification:** Accurate insurance verification at the outset ensures that services provided are covered, reducing the likelihood of denied claims and lost revenue.

- **Determining Financial Responsibility:** By determining a patient's coverage, deductibles, co-pays, and co-insurance, providers can accurately bill patients for their portion, enhancing the efficiency of the billing process.

Reducing Claim Denials

- **Preventative Measure:** Proper verification acts as a preventative measure against claim denials. Denials, often due to eligibility issues, are costly and time-consuming to rectify.

- **Streamlining Claim Approvals:** Accurate verification leads to cleaner claims, increasing the likelihood of first-time approval and faster reimbursements.

Enhancing Cash Flow

- **Predictability in Payments:** When insurance coverage is confirmed, and patient responsibilities are clearly delineated, payments become more predictable, enhancing overall cash flow.

- **Minimizing Delays:** Efficient verification minimizes delays in payment, both from insurance companies and patients, by reducing the need for rework and follow-ups on denied claims.

Patient Experience and Financial Transparency

- **Building Trust:** Clear communication about coverage and costs builds patient trust, which is crucial for patient retention and a positive reputation.

- **Reducing Financial Surprises:** When patients are informed about their financial responsibilities upfront, it reduces the likelihood of unexpected bills, enhancing patient satisfaction.

Technology's Role in Verification for Revenue Cycle Management

- **Automated Verification Tools:** Utilizing automated verification tools can speed up the process, reduce errors, and provide real-time updates on coverage changes.

- **Integration with Billing Systems:** Integrating verification systems with billing and electronic health record systems ensures that billing is accurate and reflective of the latest insurance information.

Conclusion

Insurance verification is a linchpin in the revenue cycle management of healthcare services. Its effectiveness directly impacts the financial health of healthcare organizations and the satisfaction of patients. By ensuring accurate and timely insurance verification, healthcare providers can streamline their revenue cycle, enhance cash flow, and provide a better patient experience. In this sense, insurance verification is not just a procedural necessity but a strategic asset in healthcare financial management.

9.2 Reducing Denials through Accurate Verification

The battle against insurance claim denials is a critical one in healthcare revenue cycle management. One of the most effective weapons in this fight is accurate insurance verification. It's like a navigational chart for a ship, guiding the billing process through treacherous waters to avoid the perils of denials and delays. Let's explore how accurate verification can significantly reduce the incidence of insurance denials.

Root Causes of Claim Denials

- **Eligibility Issues:** Many denials stem from eligibility issues, such as services not covered under a patient's insurance plan or lapses in coverage.

- **Data Errors:** Simple mistakes in patient data entry, incorrect policy numbers, or outdated insurance information can lead to denials.

- **Authorization Lapses:** Failing to obtain required pre-authorizations or referrals for certain procedures often results in claim rejections.

Impact of Accurate Verification

- **Preventing Eligibility-Related Denials:** Accurate verification ensures that services are eligible for coverage under the patient's current insurance plan.

- **Ensuring Up-to-Date Information:** Regularly updated verification processes help in maintaining accurate and current insurance information, reducing the risk of denials due to outdated or incorrect data.

Strategies for Accurate Verification

- **Detailed Verification Process:** Establish a thorough verification process that checks all aspects of a patient's insurance coverage, including effective dates, covered services, and benefit limits.

- **Regular Training for Staff:** Train staff regularly on the latest insurance policies and verification techniques to maintain high accuracy levels.

- **Use of Technology:** Implement advanced verification tools and software that can automate and streamline the process, reducing human error.

Double-Checking for Common Pitfalls

- **Verification at Every Visit:** Re-verify insurance at every patient visit, as insurance information and coverage can change.

- **Attention to Detail:** Pay special attention to common problem areas, such as policy numbers, patient names and dates of birth, and service codes.

Collaboration with Insurance Companies

- **Building Relationships:** Develop good working relationships with insurance companies to facilitate easier resolution of issues that may lead to denials.

- **Proactive Communication:** Proactively communicate with insurers about complex cases or unclear coverage scenarios before providing services.

Analyzing Denial Patterns

- **Data Analysis:** Regularly analyze denial data to identify patterns or common issues. Use these insights to refine verification processes.

- **Continuous Improvement:** Implement changes based on denial analysis to continuously improve the verification process and reduce future denials.

Conclusion

Reducing denials through accurate verification is a crucial aspect of maintaining a healthy revenue cycle in healthcare. It requires a combination of diligent verification practices, staff training, technological assistance, and proactive communication with insurance companies. By prioritizing accuracy in insurance verification, healthcare providers can significantly reduce the incidence of claim denials, ensuring smoother financial operations and better patient satisfaction.

9.3 Improving Cash Flow with Efficient Eligibility Checks

In the intricate world of healthcare financial management, efficient eligibility checks play a vital role in maintaining a healthy cash flow. Like a well-oiled machine, a streamlined eligibility verification process can accelerate the revenue cycle, ensuring that financial resources are optimized and maintained. Let's explore how efficient eligibility checks can lead to an improvement in cash flow within healthcare settings.

Direct Impact on Revenue Cycle

- **Speeding Up Reimbursements:** Efficient eligibility verification leads to faster claim approvals and reimbursements, reducing the time between service delivery and payment.

- **Minimizing Denials:** By accurately verifying eligibility upfront, healthcare providers can significantly reduce claim denials, a major bottleneck in cash flow.

Reducing Administrative Burdens

- **Efficiency in Operations:** Streamlining the eligibility check process frees up administrative resources, allowing staff to focus on other revenue-enhancing activities.

- **Lowering Operational Costs:** Efficient processes reduce the need for additional follow-ups and claim resubmissions, cutting down on administrative costs.

Enhanced Patient Financial Experience

- **Increased Transparency:** When patients are well-informed about their financial responsibility early in the process, it leads to timely and more reliable payments.

- **Improved Patient Trust:** Clear and upfront communication regarding coverage and costs can strengthen patient trust, leading to better patient-provider relationships and a more stable revenue flow.

Utilization of Technology

- **Automated Verification Tools:** Implementing advanced software solutions for insurance verification can provide real-time, accurate eligibility information, enhancing the speed and reliability of the process.

- **Integration with Billing Systems:** Seamless integration of eligibility verification systems with billing and Electronic Health Records (EHR) ensures that billing is accurate and reflective of the most current insurance information.

Proactive Eligibility Management

- **Regular Updates and Checks:** Consistently updating and verifying patient insurance information to accommodate changes in policies or coverage.

- **Anticipating Changes:** Staying ahead of potential changes in insurance plans or healthcare regulations that could affect patient eligibility and coverage.

Training and Development

- **Staff Training:** Ensuring that the staff responsible for eligibility checks are well-trained and knowledgeable about various insurance plans and verification techniques.

- **Continuous Learning:** Encouraging a culture of continuous learning and adaptation to new verification tools and methods.

Conclusion

Efficient eligibility checks are a key driver of healthy cash flow in healthcare organizations. They ensure that the revenue cycle is fast, accurate, and minimally interrupted by denials or delays in payment. By investing in efficient verification processes, healthcare providers can secure their financial health, ensuring that they continue to provide quality care without the hindrance of financial constraints.

9.4 Exercise: 10 MCQs with Answers at the End

1. **Efficient eligibility checks in healthcare can primarily:**

   A. Increase patient wait times.

   B. Lead to more claim denials.

   C. Speed up reimbursements.

   D. Complicate the billing process.

2. **How do efficient eligibility checks reduce administrative burdens?**

   A. By increasing paperwork.

   B. By freeing up resources for other activities.

   C. By complicating processes.

   D. By reducing staff efficiency.

3. **What is a direct impact of efficient eligibility checks on patient experience?**

A. Decreased understanding of financial responsibilities.

B. Longer billing cycles.

C. Increased transparency and reliability in payments.

D. More frequent billing errors.

4. **The use of automated verification tools in eligibility checks helps to:**

A. Delay the verification process.

B. Provide real-time, accurate eligibility information.

C. Increase manual work.

D. Decrease data accuracy.

5. **Why is integration of eligibility verification with billing systems important?**

A. To reduce the accuracy of billing.

B. To ensure billing is reflective of current insurance information.

C. To complicate the revenue cycle.

D. To discourage the use of technology.

6. **Proactive eligibility management involves:**

A. Ignoring changes in insurance policies.

B. Regularly updating patient insurance information.

C. Avoiding verification of patient information.

D. Decreasing communication with insurance providers.

7. **What role does staff training play in efficient eligibility checks?**

A. It's unnecessary and time-consuming.

B. It ensures staff are knowledgeable about verification techniques.

C. It encourages a reliance on outdated methods.

D. It decreases the efficiency of the verification process.

8. **Efficient eligibility checks impact cash flow by:**

A. Slowing down the revenue cycle.

B. Increasing claim denials.

C. Leading to faster claim approvals and reimbursements.

D. Reducing patient satisfaction.

9. **How do efficient eligibility checks affect patient-provider relationships?**

A. By creating distrust.

B. By strengthening trust through clear communication.

C. By minimizing patient interaction.

D. By increasing billing disputes.

10. **What is a benefit of continuously learning and adapting to new verification tools?**

A. Decreasing staff competence.

B. Reducing efficiency in the verification process.

C. Keeping up with changes in insurance and healthcare regulations.

D. Complicating the verification process.

Answers

1. **C. Speed up reimbursements.**

2. **B. By freeing up resources for other activities.**

3. **C. Increased transparency and reliability in payments.**

4. **B. Provide real-time, accurate eligibility information.**

5. **B. To ensure billing is reflective of current insurance information.**

6. **B. Regularly updating patient insurance information.**

7. **B. It ensures staff are knowledgeable about verification techniques.**

8. **C. Leading to faster claim approvals and reimbursements.**

9. **B. By strengthening trust through clear communication.**

10. **C. Keeping up with changes in insurance and healthcare regulations.**

Chapter 10: Training and Development for Verification Staff

10.1 Essential Skills for Verification Professionals

The competence and efficiency of verification staff are crucial in the smooth operation of the healthcare revenue cycle. Like navigators in a ship, they guide the financial aspect of patient care through the complexities of insurance policies and regulations. Let's identify the essential skills that are fundamental for professionals involved in insurance verification.

Attention to Detail

- **Accuracy in Data Entry:** Precision in entering patient information and insurance details is paramount to avoid errors that can lead to claim denials.

- **Vigilance in Reviewing Coverage:** Meticulous review of insurance coverage details to ensure accurate understanding and application.

Strong Communication Skills

- **Effective Patient Interaction:** Ability to clearly and compassionately communicate with patients regarding their insurance coverage and financial responsibilities.

- **Professional Insurance Company Liaison:** Competence in interacting with insurance company representatives to clarify coverage details and resolve issues.

Problem-Solving Abilities

- **Issue Identification and Resolution:** Skill in identifying issues in the verification process and finding effective solutions.

- **Adaptability to Changes:** Ability to adapt to changes in insurance policies and healthcare regulations.

Knowledge of Insurance Policies and Healthcare Regulations

- **Understanding of Various Insurance Plans:** Familiarity with different types of insurance plans and their specific coverage details.

- **Compliance with Healthcare Laws:** Knowledge of healthcare laws such as HIPAA, which are crucial in handling patient information.

Technological Proficiency

- **Use of Verification Software:** Proficiency in using electronic verification tools and software.

- **EHR System Navigation:** Ability to navigate Electronic Health Records (EHR) systems for accessing and updating patient information.

Organizational Skills

- **Effective Time Management:** Ability to manage time effectively to handle the high volume of verification tasks.

- **Prioritization of Tasks:** Skill in prioritizing tasks based on urgency and importance.

Continuous Learning and Development

- **Staying Informed:** Commitment to staying informed about the latest developments in healthcare insurance and technology.

- **Engagement in Ongoing Training:** Willingness to participate in ongoing training and professional development opportunities.

Customer Service Orientation

- **Patient-Centered Approach:** Focusing on patient needs and satisfaction in all interactions and processes.

- **Empathy and Understanding:** Demonstrating empathy and understanding towards patient concerns and anxieties related to insurance and healthcare costs.

Conclusion

Professionals in insurance verification play a key role in the healthcare revenue cycle, and equipping them with these essential skills is vital for the success of healthcare organizations. By fostering these competencies, verification staff can efficiently navigate the complexities of insurance verification, contributing to improved revenue cycle management, patient satisfaction, and overall operational efficiency.

10.2 Developing a Training Program for Staff

Creating a comprehensive training program for insurance verification staff is a crucial investment in the efficiency and effectiveness of healthcare operations. Think of it as equipping your team with the best tools and maps for a successful journey in the complex world of healthcare finance. Here's a guide to developing a training program that empowers your staff with the necessary skills and knowledge.

Assess Training Needs

- **Identify Skill Gaps:** Conduct an assessment to identify the specific areas where your staff needs improvement or additional knowledge.

- **Stay Current:** Ensure that the training program addresses the latest trends and changes in healthcare insurance, technology, and regulations.

Create a Structured Training Curriculum

- **Foundation Training:** Start with basic training on healthcare systems, insurance types, and key medical billing terminologies.

- **Specialized Modules:** Develop modules focusing on specific aspects like understanding different insurance plans, the nuances of eligibility and benefits, and compliance with laws like HIPAA.

- **Hands-On Training:** Include practical, scenario-based training to simulate real-life insurance verification challenges.

Utilize a Variety of Training Methods

- **Interactive Workshops:** Conduct workshops and seminars that encourage active participation and discussion.

- **Online Learning:** Leverage online courses and webinars that staff can attend remotely at their convenience.

- **In-House Training Sessions:** Regular in-house training sessions led by experienced professionals or external experts.

Regular Updates and Refreshers

- **Ongoing Education:** Provide regular update sessions to keep staff informed about changes in insurance policies, healthcare laws, and technology.

- **Refresher Courses:** Schedule periodic refresher courses to reinforce knowledge and update skills.

Incorporate Technology Training

- **Software Proficiency:** Train staff on the use of specific insurance verification software, electronic health record systems, and other relevant technology tools.

- **Data Security:** Emphasize the importance of data security and privacy in all technological training.

Evaluate and Adapt the Training Program

- **Feedback Mechanism:** Implement a feedback system to gather insights from staff about the effectiveness of the training program.

- **Continuous Improvement:** Regularly review and update the training curriculum based on feedback, performance metrics, and evolving industry standards.

Mentorship and Support

- **Mentorship Programs:** Pair less experienced staff with seasoned mentors for ongoing guidance and support.

- **Supportive Environment:** Foster a culture that encourages continuous learning and professional development.

Conclusion

A well-structured and dynamic training program is essential for empowering insurance verification staff with the skills and knowledge needed to navigate the complexities of healthcare billing and insurance. Through continuous learning, practical training, and supportive mentorship, staff can develop the proficiency required to manage insurance verification efficiently and effectively, contributing to the overall success and sustainability of healthcare operations.

10.3 Continuing Education and Certification

In the ever-evolving field of healthcare, particularly in areas like insurance verification, continuing education and certification play a vital role. They are akin to navigational updates for a pilot, ensuring that the skills and knowledge of healthcare professionals remain current and effective. Let's explore how continuing education and certification can benefit insurance verification staff and the overall healthcare system.

Importance of Continuing Education

- **Staying Updated:** Healthcare regulations, insurance policies, and technology are constantly changing. Continuing education helps staff stay informed about these changes, ensuring they are equipped to handle new challenges.

- **Enhancing Skills:** Ongoing education provides opportunities for staff to enhance their skills and knowledge, leading to improved job performance and patient satisfaction.

Types of Continuing Education

- **Workshops and Seminars:** Regular workshops or seminars on the latest trends in healthcare insurance, changes in laws, and new verification technologies.

- **Online Courses and Webinars:** Participation in online courses and webinars that focus on specific areas of healthcare billing and insurance verification.

- **Professional Conferences:** Attendance at professional conferences offers exposure to a broader range of topics and networking opportunities with peers and experts.

Role of Certification

- **Professional Recognition:** Certification provides professional recognition and validation of an individual's expertise in insurance verification and healthcare billing.

- **Career Advancement:** Certified professionals often have more opportunities for career advancement and may be viewed as more valuable assets by their employers.

Certification Programs

- **Certified Healthcare Access Associate (CHAA):** A certification that focuses on patient access services, including insurance verification.

- **Certified Professional Coder (CPC):** A certification for medical coders, including aspects of insurance verification and compliance.

- **Customized In-House Certification:** Some healthcare organizations develop their own certification programs tailored to their specific processes and needs.

Implementing a Continuing Education Program

- **Incentives for Education:** Offering incentives for staff to pursue continuing education and certification, such as tuition reimbursement or time off for studying.

- **Integrating Education in Career Development:** Making continuing education and certification a part of career development plans for staff.

Measuring the Impact

- **Performance Metrics:** Assess the impact of continuing education and certification on performance metrics like accuracy in verification, claim denial rates, and patient satisfaction.

- **Feedback from Staff:** Solicit feedback from staff on the effectiveness of the education and training programs in enhancing their work processes and knowledge.

Conclusion

Continuing education and certification are crucial in maintaining a high standard of expertise in insurance verification, adapting to the dynamic healthcare landscape. By investing in these areas, healthcare organizations can ensure their staff are well-equipped to handle the complexities of healthcare billing and insurance, ultimately leading to better patient care and more efficient operations.

10.4 Exercise: 10 MCQs with Answers at the End

1. **Continuing education for insurance verification staff is important because:**

   A. It's a legal requirement.

   B. It helps them stay updated on industry changes.

   C. It reduces their workload.

   D. It eliminates the need for technology.

2. **Which certification focuses on patient access services, including insurance verification?**

   A. Certified Professional Coder (CPC)

   B. Certified Healthcare Access Associate (CHAA)

   C. Certified Medical Assistant (CMA)

   D. Certified Insurance Specialist (CIS)

3. **Online courses and webinars for insurance verification staff:**

   A. Are unnecessary.

   B. Provide flexibility and convenience in learning.

C. Are only for new employees.

D. Decrease knowledge and skills.

4. **The role of certification in insurance verification includes:**

A. Decreasing professional standards.

B. Providing professional recognition and validating expertise.

C. Limiting career opportunities.

D. Making the job more challenging.

5. **Attending professional conferences benefits insurance verification staff by:**

A. Only providing a break from work.

B. Reducing their knowledge base.

C. Offering exposure to a range of topics and networking opportunities.

D. Increasing their workload.

6. **Implementing a continuing education program in a healthcare setting can involve:**

A. Discouraging staff from learning.

B. Offering incentives for educational advancement.

C. Ignoring industry changes.

D. Limiting access to new information.

7. **What impact does certification have on a healthcare professional's career?**

A. It has no Impact.

B. It can lead to more opportunities for career advancement.

C. It decreases their credibility.

D. It restricts their job roles.

8. **Customized in-house certification programs are:**

A. Rarely beneficial.

B. Tailored to specific organizational needs and processes.

C. Prohibited by law.

D. Designed to reduce staff efficiency.

9. **How should the impact of continuing education be measured in healthcare?**

A. By the increase in staff complaints.

B. Through performance metrics and staff feedback.

C. It should not be measured.

D. Solely by the cost of training.

10. **Why are workshops and seminars crucial in continuing education?**

A. They only serve as social events.

B. They are not as effective as online courses.

C. They encourage active participation and discussion on relevant topics.

D. They are legally required every month.

Answers

1. **B. It helps them stay updated on industry changes.**
2. **B. Certified Healthcare Access Associate (CHAA)**
3. **B. Provide flexibility and convenience in learning.**
4. **B. Providing professional recognition and validating expertise.**
5. **C. Offering exposure to a range of topics and networking opportunities.**
6. **B. Offering incentives for educational advancement.**
7. **B. It can lead to more opportunities for career advancement.**
8. **B. Tailored to specific organizational needs and processes.**
9. **B. Through performance metrics and staff feedback.**

10. **C. They encourage active participation and discussion on relevant topics.**

Chapter 11: Outsourcing Insurance Verification

11.1 Pros and Cons of Outsourcing

Outsourcing insurance verification can be likened to a strategic partnership in business. It involves delegating this crucial function to external specialists. Like any significant business decision, outsourcing comes with its own set of advantages and challenges. Let's examine the pros and cons of this approach.

Pros of Outsourcing Insurance Verification

1. **Cost Efficiency:** Outsourcing can be more cost-effective than maintaining an in-house team, especially for smaller practices that cannot afford a dedicated verification staff.

2. **Expertise and Specialization:** Outsourced providers often have specialized knowledge and expertise in insurance verification, leading to higher accuracy and efficiency.

3. **Focus on Core Activities:** It allows healthcare providers to focus on their core activities – patient care – by reducing the burden of administrative tasks.

4. **Scalability:** Outsourcing offers scalability, allowing healthcare providers to handle fluctuating volumes of verification tasks without the need for additional staffing.

5. **Technological Advantages:** Outsourced companies may have access to advanced verification tools and technologies that some healthcare practices might not possess.

Cons of Outsourcing Insurance Verification

1. **Loss of Direct Control:** Outsourcing means relinquishing some level of control over the verification process, which can be a concern for some providers.

2. **Potential for Miscommunication:** Working with an external party can sometimes lead to communication challenges, especially if they are not fully integrated with the healthcare provider's systems and processes.

3. **Privacy and Security Concerns:** There's a need to ensure that the outsourced partner adheres strictly to patient privacy laws and regulations, like HIPAA.

4. **Dependency on the Vendor:** Relying on an external party creates a dependency, which could be risky if the vendor faces operational issues or discontinues their services.

5. **Quality Variation:** The quality of services can vary among different outsourcing providers, requiring thorough research and vetting to choose the right partner.

Balancing the Decision

- **Cost-Benefit Analysis:** Conduct a thorough cost-benefit analysis to determine if outsourcing offers tangible advantages over an in-house team.

- **Vendor Selection:** Carefully select a vendor with a proven track record, positive references, and robust data security measures.

- **Contract and Agreement:** Ensure that the contract with the outsourcing company includes clear terms regarding service levels, data privacy, and compliance with healthcare regulations.

Conclusion

Outsourcing insurance verification can offer significant benefits, including cost savings and access to specialized expertise. However, it requires careful consideration of the potential drawbacks, such as loss of control and privacy concerns. Healthcare providers should weigh these factors carefully to decide whether outsourcing aligns with their operational goals and patient care standards.

11.2 Selecting an Outsourcing Partner

Choosing the right outsourcing partner for insurance verification is a crucial decision for healthcare providers, much like selecting a co-pilot for a complex flight. The right partner can streamline your insurance verification process, enhance efficiency, and improve patient satisfaction. Here are key considerations for selecting an appropriate outsourcing partner:

1. Expertise and Experience

- **Industry Knowledge:** Look for a partner with extensive knowledge of healthcare insurance verification and a deep understanding of different insurance plans and regulations.

- **Proven Track Record:** Evaluate their history and experience in handling verification for similar healthcare providers.

2. Compliance and Security

- **HIPAA Compliance:** Ensure the outsourcing partner is fully compliant with HIPAA and other relevant privacy laws.

- **Data Security:** Assess their data security measures and protocols to protect sensitive patient information.

3. Technology and Infrastructure

- **Advanced Tools:** Check if the partner uses advanced verification tools and technologies that can integrate with your existing systems.

- **Infrastructure Reliability:** Evaluate their infrastructure and technology capabilities to ensure they can handle your verification volume and complexity.

4. Quality of Service

- **Accuracy and Efficiency:** Assess their track record for accuracy in verification and efficiency in processing.

- **Service Level Agreements (SLAs):** Look for clear SLAs that outline the quality and timelines of services to be provided.

5. Communication and Support

- **Effective Communication:** Choose a partner that values and practices clear, consistent communication.

- **Support Availability:** Ensure they offer adequate support and have mechanisms for resolving issues swiftly.

6. Flexibility and Scalability

- **Adaptability:** The partner should be flexible in adapting to your specific needs and changes in healthcare policies.

- **Scalability:** They should be able to scale their services in response to your growth or changing needs.

7. Cost-Effectiveness

- **Transparent Pricing:** Look for transparent pricing models that align with your budget and offer good value for money.

- **Return on Investment:** Consider the potential return on investment, balancing cost savings with the quality of services provided.

8. References and Reviews

- **Client Feedback:** Seek feedback from current or past clients to gauge their satisfaction and experience with the outsourcing partner.

- **Reputation:** Research their reputation in the industry through reviews, testimonials, and industry forums.

9. Cultural Fit

- **Alignment with Values:** The partner should align with your organization's values, particularly regarding patient care and service.

10. Trial Period and Evaluation

- **Pilot Project:** Consider starting with a pilot project to evaluate their services before committing to a long-term contract.

- **Performance Evaluation:** Set benchmarks for performance evaluation during the trial period.

Conclusion

Selecting an outsourcing partner for insurance verification is a decision that requires careful consideration of various factors, including expertise, compliance, technology, and service quality. By thoroughly vetting potential partners against these criteria, healthcare providers can establish a fruitful partnership that enhances their revenue cycle management and overall patient care services.

11.3 Managing Outsourced Verification Processes

Effectively managing outsourced verification processes is akin to steering a ship in collaboration with a trusted ally. It requires clear communication, ongoing oversight, and strategic coordination to ensure that the outsourced functions align with the healthcare provider's standards and expectations. Let's explore how to manage these processes effectively.

Establishing Clear Communication Channels

- **Regular Check-ins:** Schedule regular meetings or calls with the outsourcing partner to discuss performance, challenges, and updates.

- **Point of Contact:** Designate specific individuals within your organization and the outsourcing company as primary contacts to streamline communication.

Setting and Monitoring Key Performance Indicators (KPIs)

- **Define KPIs:** Establish clear KPIs such as accuracy rates, turnaround times, and patient satisfaction levels to measure the performance of the outsourcing partner.

- **Regular Reporting:** Ensure that the outsourcing partner provides regular reports against these KPIs, allowing for continuous monitoring of their performance.

Ensuring Quality Control

- **Random Audits:** Conduct random audits of the work done by the outsourcing partner to ensure adherence to quality standards.

- **Feedback Mechanism:** Implement a system for feedback where discrepancies or issues are promptly communicated and addressed.

Integrating Systems and Processes

- **Technological Integration:** Where possible, integrate your systems with those of the outsourcing partner for seamless data exchange and better coordination.

- **Process Alignment:** Ensure that the outsourced processes are aligned with your internal procedures, especially regarding patient data handling and privacy.

Training and Knowledge Sharing

- **Joint Training Sessions:** Consider joint training sessions on specific aspects of insurance verification, updates in healthcare laws, or new software tools.

- **Shared Best Practices:** Encourage the sharing of best practices and insights between your team and the outsourcing partner.

Handling Compliance and Security

- **Regular Compliance Checks:** Regularly review the outsourcing partner's adherence to compliance standards, especially HIPAA and other relevant healthcare regulations.

- **Data Security:** Continuously monitor the data security measures in place to protect patient information.

Managing Change

- **Adaptability to Changes:** Be prepared to adapt and modify the agreement with the outsourcing partner in response to changes in healthcare regulations, insurance policies, or your own operational needs.

- **Contingency Planning:** Have contingency plans in place in case of service disruption or termination of the outsourcing agreement.

Building a Partnership

- **Long-Term Relationship:** Foster a sense of partnership rather than a transactional relationship, focusing on mutual growth and improvement.

- **Openness to Feedback:** Be open to receiving and acting on feedback from the outsourcing partner regarding potential improvements in processes or coordination.

Conclusion

Managing outsourced verification processes requires a balanced approach of oversight, collaboration, and continuous improvement. By actively engaging with the outsourcing partner, setting clear performance metrics, and ensuring quality and compliance, healthcare providers can effectively manage these processes, leading to enhanced efficiency, reduced costs, and improved patient satisfaction.

11.4 Exercise: 10 MCQs with Answers at the End

1. **Effective management of outsourced verification processes includes:**

   A. Ignoring the outsourced team's performance.

   B. Regularly scheduling check-ins and meetings.

   C. Avoiding feedback mechanisms.

   D. Isolating the outsourced team from internal processes.

2. **Key Performance Indicators (KPIs) for outsourced verification processes are important because they:**

   A. Complicate the working relationship.

   B. Measure the performance of the outsourcing partner.

   C. Are irrelevant to the quality of service.

   D. Decrease operational transparency.

3. **Quality control in outsourced verification can be ensured by:**

A. Trusting the outsourcing partner blindly.

B. Conducting random audits and having a feedback mechanism.

C. Eliminating all checks and balances.

D. Decreasing communication frequency.

4. **Technological integration with an outsourcing partner helps in:**

A. Reducing data accuracy.

B. Increasing data breaches.

C. Streamlining data exchange and coordination.

D. Complicating processes unnecessarily.

5. **The primary role of regular compliance checks with an outsourcing partner is to:**

A. Increase paperwork.

B. Ensure adherence to healthcare regulations.

C. Make the process more bureaucratic.

D. Confuse the outsourcing partner.

6. **Joint training sessions with an outsourcing partner are beneficial for:**

A. Reducing the effectiveness of processes.

B. Sharing best practices and insights.

C. Creating competition between teams.

D. Avoiding updates on healthcare laws.

7. **In managing outsourced verification processes, contingency planning is important for:**

A. Ignoring potential risks.

B. Preparing for service disruption or changes.

C. Creating unnecessary panic.

D. Making the process more expensive.

8. **Regular reporting and monitoring of KPIs by an outsourcing partner:**

A. Is not necessary.

B. Allows for continuous performance evaluation.

C. Should be avoided to save time.

D. Has no impact on service quality.

9. **Adaptability in the outsourcing agreement is crucial due to:**

A. The static nature of healthcare regulations.

B. Changes in healthcare regulations, insurance policies, or operational needs.

C. The preference for a rigid structure.

D. The unimportance of staying current.

10. **A successful partnership with an outsourcing partner is characterized by:**

A. A transactional relationship.

B. Mutual growth and improvement.

C. Limited communication.

D. Avoiding feedback.

Answers

1. **B. Regularly scheduling check-ins and meetings.**

2. **B. Measure the performance of the outsourcing partner.**

3. **B. Conducting random audits and having a feedback mechanism.**

4. **C. Streamlining data exchange and coordination.**

5. **B. Ensure adherence to healthcare regulations.**

6. **B. Sharing best practices and insights.**

7. **B. Preparing for service disruption or changes.**

8. **B. Allows for continuous performance evaluation.**

9. **B. Changes in healthcare regulations, insurance policies, or operational needs.**

10. **B. Mutual growth and improvement.**

Chapter 12: Insurance Verification for Elective Procedures

12.1 Specific Considerations for Elective Care

Insurance verification for elective procedures, which are typically non-emergency and often optional, involves a distinct set of considerations compared to emergency or medically necessary care. These procedures, ranging from cosmetic surgeries to certain orthopedic operations, require a nuanced approach in insurance verification. Let's explore the specific considerations that healthcare providers must keep in mind for elective care.

Understanding Coverage Nuances

- **Variable Insurance Coverage:** Elective procedures often have different levels of coverage depending on the patient's insurance plan. Some may not be covered at all, especially if deemed cosmetic or not medically necessary.

- **Pre-Authorization Requirements:** Many insurance plans require pre-authorization for elective procedures to determine if they are covered.

Communicating with Patients

- **Clear Explanation of Coverage:** It is essential to clearly communicate to patients what is and isn't covered by their insurance for an elective procedure.

- **Discussion of Potential Costs:** Patients should be informed about potential out-of-pocket costs, including deductibles, co-pays, and any expenses not covered by insurance.

Documentation and Rationale

- **Medical Necessity Documentation:** In cases where an elective procedure might be covered due to medical necessity, thorough documentation justifying the procedure is crucial.

- **Rationale for the Procedure:** Providing a clear rationale for the procedure can assist in obtaining insurance authorization and coverage.

Financial Agreements and Deposits

- **Financial Agreements:** Have clear financial agreements in place, outlining the patient's financial responsibilities.

- **Deposits for Non-Covered Services:** For procedures not covered by insurance, consider requiring deposits or full payment in advance.

Handling Denials and Appeals

- **Proactive Management of Denials:** Be prepared to handle insurance denials for elective procedures, including submitting appeals with adequate supporting documentation.

- **Patient Advocacy:** Assist patients in navigating the appeals process if a claim for an elective procedure is denied.

Insurance Liaison

- **Direct Communication with Insurers:** Maintain direct communication with insurance companies to clarify coverage details and authorization requirements for elective procedures.

- **Up-to-Date Knowledge:** Stay informed about changes in insurance policies regarding elective procedures.

Conclusion

Verification of insurance for elective procedures demands a detailed and patient-centric approach. Understanding the intricacies of insurance coverage, communicating effectively with patients, and ensuring proper documentation and rationale are key to managing the verification process for elective care. By doing so, healthcare providers can minimize financial surprises for patients and ensure a smoother administrative process.

12.2 Pre-Authorization Processes

In the realm of healthcare, pre-authorization for certain procedures, especially elective ones, is a critical step in the insurance verification process. It's like obtaining a key that unlocks the door to insurance coverage. Pre-authorization ensures that the proposed medical service or procedure is covered under the patient's insurance plan and is medically necessary. Let's delve into the essential aspects of pre-authorization processes.

Understanding Pre-Authorization

- **Definition:** Pre-authorization is a requirement by an insurance company or payer that a healthcare provider obtains approval before performing a specific service to ensure coverage.

- **Purpose:** It's designed to prevent unnecessary procedures and control healthcare costs.

Steps in the Pre-Authorization Process

1. **Verifying the Requirement:** Determine if the proposed procedure requires pre-authorization as per the patient's insurance policy.

2. **Gathering Necessary Information:** Collect all relevant patient information and details about the planned procedure, including medical necessity documentation.

3. **Submitting the Request:** Fill out the pre-authorization request form provided by the insurance company and submit it along with any required supporting documentation, such as medical records or test results.

4. **Follow-Up:** Regularly follow up with the insurance company to check the status of the authorization request.

Documentation for Pre-Authorization

- **Clinical Information:** Provide detailed clinical information, including diagnosis, proposed treatment plan, and expected outcomes.

- **Evidence of Medical Necessity:** Present evidence that the procedure is medically necessary and is the most appropriate treatment option.

Handling Denials in Pre-Authorization

- **Review Denial Reasons:** Carefully review the reasons for any denial and address them specifically in an appeal.

- **Appeal Process:** Understand the insurance company's appeal process and submit a well-documented appeal if necessary.

Communication with Patients

- **Informing Patients:** Keep patients informed throughout the pre-authorization process. Let them know about any potential delays or issues.

- **Discussing Alternatives:** If pre-authorization is denied, discuss alternative treatments or options with the patient.

Best Practices

- **Timely Submission:** Submit pre-authorization requests well in advance of the scheduled procedure to avoid delays.

- **Training Staff:** Ensure staff are well-trained in the pre-authorization process and understand the nuances of different insurance policies.

- **Record Keeping:** Keep detailed records of all communications and submissions related to pre-authorization requests.

Conclusion

The pre-authorization process is a critical component in managing healthcare procedures, particularly elective ones. By effectively navigating this process, healthcare providers can ensure that the necessary treatments are approved by insurance companies, thereby safeguarding both the financial interests of the practice and the healthcare needs of the patients.

12.3 Managing Patient Financial Responsibility

Effectively managing patient financial responsibility in the context of elective procedures is a crucial aspect of healthcare administration. It's akin to guiding patients through a financial landscape, ensuring they understand their obligations and are prepared for potential expenses. This management is vital for maintaining transparency, patient satisfaction, and the financial health of the healthcare practice.

Clarifying Insurance Coverage and Patient Liability

- **Upfront Discussions:** Initiate clear, upfront discussions with patients about what their insurance covers and what costs they are responsible for.

- **Detailed Breakdown:** Provide a detailed breakdown of potential costs, including deductibles, co-pays, and non-covered services.

Educating Patients on Insurance Limitations

- **Insurance Limitations:** Educate patients on the limitations of their insurance coverage, especially for elective procedures, which may not be fully covered.

- **Alternative Payment Options:** Discuss alternative payment options for services not covered by insurance, such as payment plans or financial assistance programs.

Establishing Financial Policies

- **Transparent Policies:** Develop and communicate transparent financial policies regarding patient responsibilities for elective procedures.

- **Consent and Agreement:** Obtain written consent and agreement from patients acknowledging their understanding and acceptance of their financial responsibilities.

Utilizing Estimates and Pre-Authorization

- **Cost Estimates:** Provide patients with estimates of their potential financial responsibility based on pre-authorization information and insurance coverage details.

- **Incorporating Pre-Authorization:** Use the pre-authorization process to obtain a clearer understanding of what the insurance will cover and communicate this to the patient.

Implementing Financial Counseling

- **Financial Counseling Services:** Offer financial counseling services to help patients navigate their insurance coverage and understand their financial obligations.

- **Payment Plan Options:** Discuss and arrange payment plan options for patients who might struggle with upfront payments.

Proactive Communication

- **Regular Updates:** Keep patients informed about any changes or updates regarding their insurance coverage or financial responsibility.

- **Responsive Service:** Ensure that staff are available to answer any financial questions or concerns patients may have.

Technology Integration

- **Billing Software:** Utilize advanced billing software that can provide accurate and clear billing statements, helping patients understand their charges.

- **Online Portals:** Offer online portals where patients can view their billing information, insurance coverage details, and make payments.

Conclusion

Managing patient financial responsibility, particularly for elective procedures, requires clear communication, transparency, and compassionate guidance. By effectively educating patients about their financial obligations and offering support through financial counseling and flexible payment options, healthcare providers can enhance patient trust, reduce financial misunderstandings, and ensure a smoother financial experience for both the patient and the practice.

12.4 Exercise: 10 MCQs with Answers at the End

1. **Why is clarifying insurance coverage and patient liability important in elective procedures?**

A. To increase the complexity of billing.

B. To ensure patient understanding of financial responsibilities.

C. To discourage patients from elective procedures.

D. To complicate insurance claims.

2. **What role does financial counseling play in managing patient financial responsibility?**

A. Confuses patients about their insurance.

B. Helps patients navigate insurance coverage and understand their obligations.

C. Reduces the accuracy of billing statements.

D. Increases the cost of healthcare services.

3. **Transparent financial policies for elective procedures are crucial because they:**

A. Minimize clear communication with patients.

B. Help patients understand their financial obligations.

C. Are irrelevant to the billing process.

D. Increase the likelihood of insurance fraud.

4. **Providing patients with cost estimates for elective procedures is important to:**

A. Create confusion about potential expenses.

B. Give patients an idea of potential financial responsibility.

C. Discourage them from receiving care.

D. Overcharge for services.

5. **What is a significant aspect of managing patient financial responsibility?**

A. Avoiding discussions about costs.

B. Educating patients on insurance limitations.

C. Providing inaccurate cost estimates.

D. Eliminating all payment options.

6. **Utilizing billing software in managing patient financial responsibility helps by:**

A. Decreasing transparency in billing.

B. Providing accurate and clear billing statements.

C. Complicating the payment process.

D. Ignoring insurance coverage details.

7. **The use of online portals in managing patient financial responsibility allows patients to:**

A. Avoid paying their bills.

B. View billing information and make payments online.

C. Become confused about their charges.

D. Dispute all charges regardless of accuracy.

8. **Regular updates and proactive communication about financial responsibilities ensure that:**

A. Patients are confused about their bills.

B. Patients remain informed about changes in coverage or costs.

C. There are more disputes over billing.

D. Patients ignore their financial obligations.

9. **Obtaining written consent and agreement from patients regarding their financial responsibilities helps to:**

A. Disregard the importance of patient understanding.

B. Ensure there is mutual understanding and agreement.

C. Overwhelm patients with paperwork.

D. Increase legal disputes with patients.

10. **Payment plan options for elective procedures are offered to:**

A. Complicate the payment process.

B. Help patients manage upfront payments for uncovered services.

C. Discourage patients from paying.

D. Increase the overall cost of care.

Answers

1. **B. To ensure patient understanding of financial responsibilities.**

2. **B. Helps patients navigate insurance coverage and understand their obligations.**

3. **B. Help patients understand their financial obligations.**

4. **B. Give patients an idea of potential financial responsibility.**

5. **B. Educating patients on insurance limitations.**

6. **B. Providing accurate and clear billing statements.**

7. **B. View billing information and make payments online.**

8. **B. Patients remain informed about changes in coverage or costs.**

9. **B. Ensure there is mutual understanding and agreement.**

10. **B. Help patients manage upfront payments for uncovered services.**

Chapter 13: Advanced Verification Techniques

13.1 Utilizing Analytics in Verification

Incorporating analytics into the insurance verification process is like using advanced navigation tools to chart a course through complex waters. It involves leveraging data analysis and predictive modeling to enhance the accuracy and efficiency of insurance verification. Let's explore how analytics can be utilized in this crucial aspect of healthcare administration.

Data-Driven Verification

- **Analyzing Trends:** Use data analytics to identify trends in insurance claims and denials, which can inform more effective verification strategies.

- **Predictive Modeling:** Implement predictive models to foresee common issues in insurance verification, such as coverage lapses or eligibility problems.

Enhanced Accuracy and Efficiency

- **Reducing Errors:** Analytics can help pinpoint areas prone to errors, enabling targeted improvements in the verification process.

- **Streamlining Processes:** By analyzing workflow data, healthcare providers can streamline their verification processes for greater efficiency.

Risk Assessment and Management

- **Identifying High-Risk Areas:** Utilize analytics to identify high-risk factors in the verification process, such as specific procedures or patient demographics with higher denial rates.

- **Proactive Risk Management:** Develop strategies to proactively address these risks before they impact the revenue cycle.

Customizing Patient Communication

- **Targeted Patient Education:** Use data insights to customize communication with patients, focusing on areas where they are more likely to encounter issues with their insurance.

- **Improving Patient Experience:** By anticipating and addressing insurance-related concerns, healthcare providers can enhance the overall patient experience.

Integrating with Other Systems

- **EHR Integration:** Integrate analytics tools with Electronic Health Records (EHR) and other healthcare systems for a more holistic approach to patient data management.

- **Real-Time Data Access:** Ensure real-time access to data, enabling immediate and informed decisions in the verification process.

Continuous Learning and Improvement

- **Feedback Loop:** Create a feedback loop where outcomes from the verification process inform ongoing analytics, leading to continuous improvement.

- **Staff Training:** Train staff to understand and utilize analytics in their daily verification tasks effectively.

Compliance Monitoring

- **Regulatory Compliance:** Use analytics to monitor compliance with healthcare regulations, such as HIPAA, in the verification process.

- **Audit Trails:** Maintain detailed audit trails for accountability and quality control.

Conclusion

Utilizing analytics in insurance verification transforms it from a reactive to a proactive, data-driven process. By harnessing the power of data, healthcare providers can anticipate issues, streamline workflows, enhance patient communication, and continuously improve their verification processes. This approach not only increases the efficiency and accuracy of insurance verification but also contributes to the overall financial health and patient satisfaction within the healthcare system.

13.2 Innovative Approaches to Verification

In the dynamic world of healthcare, embracing innovative approaches to insurance verification is akin to charting new territories with advanced tools and strategies. These innovative methods aim to enhance accuracy, efficiency, and patient satisfaction. Let's explore some of the cutting-edge approaches reshaping the insurance verification landscape.

Integration of Artificial Intelligence (AI) and Machine Learning

- **Automated Verification:** Utilize AI algorithms to automate repetitive aspects of the verification process, thereby increasing speed and reducing human error.

- **Predictive Analysis:** Implement machine learning to analyze patterns in insurance claims and denials, predicting potential issues before they arise.

Blockchain Technology

- **Secure Data Management:** Explore the use of blockchain for secure and transparent management of patient insurance data, enhancing data integrity and privacy.

- **Smart Contracts:** Implement blockchain-based smart contracts to automate verification and authorization processes, reducing manual intervention and streamlining operations.

Mobile Technology and Apps

- **Patient-Facing Apps:** Develop or adopt mobile applications that allow patients to upload their insurance information, check coverage details, and receive real-time updates about their verification status.

- **QR Code Scanning:** Utilize QR code scanning for quick retrieval and verification of patient insurance details.

Telehealth Integration

- **Verification for Remote Services:** Adapt verification processes to accommodate the nuances of telehealth services, ensuring seamless coverage verification for remote care.

- **Virtual Assistance:** Employ virtual assistants or chatbots to guide patients through the insurance verification process online.

Cloud-Based Solutions

- **Centralized Data Access:** Leverage cloud-based platforms for centralized access to patient insurance information, enhancing collaboration and accessibility.

- **Real-Time Updates:** Ensure that cloud solutions provide real-time updates on insurance policies and coverage changes.

Self-Service Kiosks

- **Automated Patient Check-In:** Implement self-service kiosks at healthcare facilities where patients can independently verify their insurance information upon arrival.

- **Integration with Internal Systems:** Ensure kiosks are integrated with the healthcare provider's internal systems for immediate update and processing of verification data.

Collaborative Platforms

- **Inter-Provider Platforms:** Participate in or develop collaborative platforms that allow different healthcare providers to share and access insurance verification information, reducing duplication of effort.

- **Payer Collaboration:** Work closely with insurance payers to develop integrated systems and protocols for more efficient verification processes.

Personalized Patient Communication Tools

- **Customized Alerts and Reminders:** Utilize tools that send personalized alerts and reminders to patients about pending verifications or required documentation.

- **Interactive Patient Portals:** Enhance patient portals with interactive features that allow patients to view and manage their insurance verification status.

Conclusion

Incorporating innovative approaches in insurance verification is about harnessing the power of technology and collaboration to transform a traditionally administrative process into a more efficient, secure, and patient-friendly experience. By adopting these advanced techniques, healthcare providers can stay ahead in the rapidly evolving landscape of healthcare administration, offering improved services and patient care.

13.3 Addressing Complex Verification Scenarios

In the multifaceted world of healthcare insurance, complex verification scenarios are not uncommon. These situations require a combination of expertise, adaptability, and strategic problem-solving. Like navigating through a labyrinth, healthcare providers must find effective ways to address these challenging scenarios. Let's delve into strategies for handling complex insurance verification cases.

Identifying Complex Scenarios

- **Multiple Insurance Plans:** Patients with more than one insurance plan, such as primary and secondary coverage, pose a challenge in determining coordination of benefits.

- **Out-of-State Insurance:** Verifying coverage for patients with insurance plans from a different state, which may have different rules and coverage limits.

- **High-Cost Procedures:** Procedures with high costs or that fall under specialized care, like transplants or certain cancer treatments, often require detailed verification and pre-authorization.

Strategies for Handling Complexity

1. **Detailed Review and Documentation:** Conduct a thorough review of all pertinent documents and details. Maintain meticulous records of all interactions and submissions.

2. **Expert Consultation:** Consult with experts or specialized team members who have experience dealing with similar complex scenarios.

3. **Direct Communication with Insurance Companies:** In cases of ambiguity or complexity, directly communicate with insurance providers to clarify coverage details and requirements.

4. **Use of Advanced Verification Tools:** Leverage sophisticated insurance verification tools that can handle complex scenarios, such as software that can manage multiple insurance plans or track high-cost procedures.

5. **Training on Specific Scenarios:** Provide specialized training to staff on handling complex verification cases, including scenario-based training and workshops.

6. **Patient Education and Communication:** Clearly communicate with patients about the complexity of their situation. Keep them informed throughout the verification process, especially regarding potential delays or issues.

Navigating Policy Changes and Exceptions

- **Staying Informed:** Stay up-to-date with changes in insurance policies that could affect complex scenarios.

- **Handling Exceptions:** Develop a protocol for handling exceptions or unusual cases, ensuring that these are managed accurately and efficiently.

Collaborative Approach

- **Interdisciplinary Collaboration:** Work collaboratively with different departments within the healthcare facility, such as billing, legal, and clinical teams, to address complex scenarios comprehensively.

- **External Partnerships:** Establish partnerships with external agencies or specialists who can provide additional support or expertise in complex verification cases.

Continuous Monitoring and Follow-Up

- **Regular Updates:** Monitor the progress of complex verifications regularly and provide updates to all relevant parties.

- **Proactive Follow-Up:** Be proactive in following up with insurance companies, especially in scenarios involving pre-authorizations or appeals.

Conclusion

Addressing complex insurance verification scenarios requires a multifaceted approach, including thorough documentation, expert consultation, direct insurer communication, and advanced tools. By adopting these strategies, healthcare providers can effectively navigate the intricacies of complex verification cases, ensuring accurate coverage determination and enhancing overall patient care and satisfaction.

13.4 Exercise: 10 MCQs with Answers at the End

1. **In complex verification scenarios involving multiple insurance plans, the main challenge is:**

   A. Determining the primary coverage.

   B. Convincing patients to choose one plan.

   C. Increasing the cost of care.

   D. Simplifying medical procedures.

2. **Why is direct communication with insurance companies important in complex verification scenarios?**

   A. To reduce the efficiency of the process.

   B. For clarity on coverage details and requirements.

   C. To avoid dealing with patients.

   D. To increase paperwork.

3. **How do advanced verification tools aid in handling complex scenarios?**

A. By complicating the verification process.

B. By managing multiple insurance plans and tracking high-cost procedures.

C. By ignoring minor details.

D. By reducing data accuracy.

4. **Expert consultation in complex verification scenarios is necessary for:**

A. Delaying the verification process.

B. Providing insight based on experience with similar cases.

C. Avoiding responsibility.

D. Increasing costs unnecessarily.

5. **A proactive follow-up in complex verification scenarios is important because it:**

A. Lengthens the verification process.

B. Ensures timely processing and resolution.

C. Creates confusion in coverage details.

D. Discourages patients from seeking care.

6. **What is the purpose of specialized training on complex verification scenarios?**

A. To confuse the staff.

B. To prepare staff to handle challenging cases effectively.

C. To limit the staff's knowledge.

D. To increase dependency on technology.

7. **In complex verification cases, detailed review and documentation are important to:**

A. Increase the workload.

B. Maintain accurate records of interactions and submissions.

C. Create unnecessary bureaucracy.

D. Complicate the verification process.

8. **Collaborative approach in managing complex scenarios involves:**

A. Working in isolation.

B. Interaction among different departments within the healthcare facility.

C. Avoiding external partnerships.

D. Reducing communication with insurance companies.

9. **Handling policy changes and exceptions in complex verification scenarios requires:**

A. Ignoring updates in insurance policies.

B. Staying informed and developing protocols for exceptions.

C. Relying on outdated information.

D. Avoiding adaptation to new scenarios.

10. **Patient education and communication in complex verification cases are key to:**

A. Misleading the patient about their coverage.

B. Keeping patients informed about potential delays or issues.

C. Overcomplicating the information given to patients.

D. Reducing transparency with patients.

Answers

1. **A. Determining the primary coverage.**

2. **B. For clarity on coverage details and requirements.**

3. **B. By managing multiple insurance plans and tracking high-cost procedures.**

4. **B. Providing insight based on experience with similar cases.**

5. **B. Ensures timely processing and resolution.**

6. **B. To prepare staff to handle challenging cases effectively.**

7. **B. Maintain accurate records of interactions and submissions.**

8. **B. Interaction among different departments within the healthcare facility.**

9. **B. Staying informed and developing protocols for exceptions.**

10. **B. Keeping patients informed about potential delays or issues.**

Chapter 14: Quality Assurance in Eligibility Verification

14.1 Implementing Quality Control Measures

Quality assurance in eligibility verification is essential for maintaining high standards of accuracy and efficiency in healthcare services. It's like ensuring every part of a machine is functioning optimally to achieve the best overall performance. Implementing effective quality control measures can significantly reduce errors, improve patient satisfaction, and enhance the financial health of the healthcare facility. Let's explore the key strategies for implementing these measures.

Regular Audits and Reviews

- **Routine Audits:** Conduct regular audits of the eligibility verification process to identify any errors or inconsistencies.

- **Performance Reviews:** Regularly review the performance of staff involved in verification to ensure adherence to best practices and protocols.

Standardization of Procedures

- **Uniform Processes:** Develop and implement standardized procedures for eligibility verification across all departments to ensure consistency and reduce errors.

- **Checklists and Guidelines:** Create comprehensive checklists and guidelines for staff to follow during the verification process.

Training and Staff Development

- **Ongoing Training:** Provide continuous training for staff on the latest insurance policies, verification techniques, and best practices.

- **Feedback Mechanisms:** Establish a system for staff to give and receive feedback on the verification process, fostering a culture of continuous improvement.

Technology Utilization

- **Verification Software:** Utilize advanced verification software that can automate certain aspects of the process and flag potential issues.

- **Data Analytics:** Apply data analytics to monitor and analyze trends in verification errors or denials, using these insights to refine processes.

Error Reporting and Management

- **Error Tracking System:** Implement a system for tracking and reporting errors in the verification process.

- **Corrective Actions:** Develop a protocol for promptly addressing any identified errors and preventing their recurrence.

Patient Communication and Feedback

- **Patient Involvement:** Involve patients in the verification process by confirming their information and coverage details.

- **Patient Feedback:** Regularly collect and analyze patient feedback on their experience with the insurance verification process.

Collaboration with Insurance Companies

- **Direct Communication:** Establish direct communication channels with insurance companies for clarifying coverage details and resolving discrepancies.

- **Joint Quality Initiatives:** Work on joint quality initiatives with insurance providers to enhance the accuracy and efficiency of the verification process.

Benchmarking and Performance Metrics

- **Industry Benchmarks:** Set benchmarks based on industry standards for eligibility verification accuracy and efficiency.

- **Performance Metrics:** Use key performance indicators (KPIs) to measure the success of the verification process and identify areas for improvement.

Continuous Quality Improvement

- **Quality Improvement Teams:** Form dedicated teams to focus on continuous quality improvement in the verification process.

- **Regular Process Evaluation:** Continually evaluate and update verification processes based on performance metrics, staff feedback, and changing industry practices.

Conclusion

Quality assurance in eligibility verification is a dynamic and ongoing process. By implementing these quality control measures, healthcare providers can enhance the accuracy and efficiency of their verification processes, leading to better patient care, reduced financial risk, and overall operational excellence.

14.2 Regular Auditing and Monitoring

Regular auditing and monitoring are integral components of quality assurance in the insurance verification process. These practices are akin to conducting regular health check-ups to ensure the system's well-being and efficiency. Through consistent evaluation, healthcare providers can identify areas for improvement, prevent errors, and maintain high standards of service. Let's delve into the strategies for effective auditing and monitoring.

Establishing a Routine Auditing Schedule

- **Frequency of Audits:** Set a regular schedule for auditing the verification process, such as monthly or quarterly, depending on the volume of patients and complexity of cases.

- **Comprehensive Audits:** Ensure that audits comprehensively review all aspects of the verification process, from initial data entry to final insurance authorization.

Key Areas to Monitor

- **Accuracy of Information:** Check for the accuracy of patient information, insurance details, and coverage verification.

- **Compliance with Policies:** Monitor compliance with internal policies and procedures, as well as external regulations like HIPAA.

- **Timeliness:** Evaluate the timeliness of the verification process, ensuring that verifications are completed within a reasonable timeframe.

Utilizing Technology for Auditing

- **Automated Tools:** Employ automated tools that can assist in monitoring the verification process, flagging errors or inconsistencies for review.

- **Data Analysis:** Use data analytics to analyze trends in verification, identifying common errors or bottlenecks.

Performance Metrics

- **Setting KPIs:** Establish Key Performance Indicators (KPIs) such as error rates, denial rates due to verification Issues, and patient satisfaction scores related to the verification process.

- **Regular Reporting:** Implement a system for regular reporting on these KPIs, allowing for ongoing assessment and improvement.

Staff Involvement and Training

- **Engaging Staff:** Involve staff in the auditing process, encouraging them to understand its importance and contribute to quality improvement.

- **Feedback and Training:** Use audit findings as a basis for staff feedback and targeted training sessions to address identified issues.

Error Correction and Process Improvement

- **Corrective Actions:** Develop a system for immediate correction of errors identified during audits.

- **Continuous Process Improvement:** Use audit results to continuously refine and improve the verification process, adapting to new challenges and changes in insurance practices.

Stakeholder Feedback

- **Patient Feedback:** Collect and analyze feedback from patients regarding their experience with the insurance verification process.

- **Insurance Provider Feedback:** Seek feedback from insurance providers on the quality and accuracy of submitted verifications.

Documentation and Record Keeping

- **Audit Records:** Maintain detailed records of all audit findings, corrective actions, and improvements made.

- **Transparency and Accountability:** Ensure transparency in the audit process, with clear documentation and accountability for all aspects of verification.

Conclusion

Regular auditing and monitoring are essential for maintaining the integrity and effectiveness of the insurance verification process. By consistently evaluating performance, correcting errors, and adapting to changes, healthcare providers can ensure high-quality service delivery, minimize financial risks, and improve patient satisfaction in their insurance verification practices.

14.3 Continuous Improvement in Verification Processes

Continuous improvement in insurance verification processes is akin to a journey of constant evolution, aiming to enhance efficiency, accuracy, and patient satisfaction. In the fast-paced and ever-changing healthcare environment, staying adaptive and proactive is key. Let's explore strategies for fostering continuous improvement in insurance verification.

Implementing a Feedback Loop

- **Feedback Collection:** Regularly gather feedback from staff involved in the verification process, as well as from patients, to identify areas for improvement.

- **Analysis and Action:** Analyze this feedback to understand underlying issues and implement actionable solutions.

Leveraging Technology for Efficiency

- **Up-to-Date Systems:** Continuously update verification software and systems to ensure they meet current needs and utilize the latest technological advancements.

- **Automation of Repetitive Tasks:** Automate repetitive aspects of the verification process to reduce human error and free up staff for more complex tasks.

Staff Training and Development

- **Ongoing Education:** Provide continuous training opportunities for staff to stay updated on the latest insurance policies, verification techniques, and technology.

- **Cross-Training:** Encourage cross-training among staff to foster a more versatile and knowledgeable team.

Process Re-evaluation and Redesign

- **Regular Review:** Routinely review the entire verification process to identify bottlenecks, inefficiencies, or outdated practices.

- **Process Redesign:** Be willing to redesign processes based on these reviews, implementing more efficient and effective methods.

Benchmarking Against Industry Standards

- **Comparative Analysis:** Regularly compare your verification process with industry standards or benchmarks to gauge performance and identify improvement areas.

- **Best Practices Adoption:** Adopt best practices from industry leaders or other healthcare organizations that demonstrate excellence in verification processes.

Data-Driven Decision Making

- **Metrics and KPIs:** Use key metrics and Key Performance Indicators (KPIs) to measure the effectiveness of the verification process over time.

- **Data Analysis:** Employ data analysis to uncover trends, patterns, and areas that require attention or improvement.

Encouraging Innovation and Creativity

- **Idea Generation:** Encourage staff to propose innovative ideas for improving the verification process.

- **Pilot Projects:** Test new approaches on a small scale through pilot projects before wider implementation.

Building a Culture of Quality

- **Quality First Mindset:** Foster a culture where quality assurance is a priority, and continuous improvement is a shared responsibility.

- **Recognition and Rewards:** Recognize and reward staff contributions towards process improvements and high-quality performance.

Collaboration and Communication

- **Interdepartmental Collaboration:** Promote collaboration between different departments (e.g., billing, clinical, administrative) to enhance the verification process.

- **Transparent Communication:** Maintain open and transparent communication regarding changes, updates, and improvements in the process.

Conclusion

Continuous improvement in insurance verification is an ongoing commitment to excellence. By incorporating feedback, utilizing technology, engaging in regular training and process re-evaluation, and fostering a culture of innovation and quality, healthcare organizations can ensure that their insurance verification processes remain effective, efficient, and aligned with the best patient care practices.

14.4 Exercise: 10 MCQs with Answers at the End

1. **What is the primary goal of continuous improvement in insurance verification processes?**

   A. To increase paperwork for staff.

   B. To enhance efficiency, accuracy, and patient satisfaction.

   C. To complicate the verification process.

   D. To reduce staff training.

2. **How does implementing a feedback loop contribute to the verification process?**

   A. By ignoring staff and patient experiences.

   B. It doesn't contribute significantly.

   C. By identifying areas for improvement based on feedback.

   D. By increasing the complexity of the process.

3. **What role does technology play in continuous improvement of verification processes?**

   A. Decreasing efficiency and accuracy.

   B. Automating repetitive tasks and updating systems.

   C. Reducing the need for staff training.

   D. Limiting access to patient information.

4. **Cross-training among staff in the verification process is beneficial because it:**

A. Decreases team versatility.

B. Reduces overall efficiency.

C. Fosters a more knowledgeable and adaptable team.

D. Is an unnecessary use of resources.

5. **Regular process re-evaluation and redesign help in:**

A. Maintaining outdated methods.

B. Identifying and addressing inefficiencies in the verification process.

C. Increasing the error rate.

D. Discouraging staff feedback.

6. **Benchmarking against industry standards in verification processes is important for:**

A. Keeping the process unchanged.

B. Gauging performance and identifying improvement areas.

C. Reducing staff morale.

D. Completely copying other organizations' processes.

7. **Data-driven decision making in verification processes involves:**

A. Ignoring all forms of data and metrics.

B. Using metrics and data analysis to measure and improve effectiveness.

C. Reducing the focus on quality.

D. Making decisions based solely on intuition.

8. **Encouraging innovation and creativity among staff in the verification process leads to:**

A. Less effective solutions.

B. Stagnation in process improvement.

C. Generation of new ideas for process enhancement.

D. Increased dependency on traditional methods.

9. **Building a culture of quality in insurance verification emphasizes:**

A. Lowering standards and expectations.

B. Prioritizing quality and shared responsibility for improvement.

C. Discouraging staff participation in quality initiatives.

D. Focusing solely on cost reduction.

10. **What is the importance of interdepartmental collaboration in improving verification processes?**

A. It creates unnecessary communication.

B. It leads to isolated working environments.

C. Enhances the process through diverse perspectives and expertise.

D. It is not important.

Answers

1. **B. To enhance efficiency, accuracy, and patient satisfaction.**
2. **C. By identifying areas for improvement based on feedback.**
3. **B. Automating repetitive tasks and updating systems.**
4. **C. Fosters a more knowledgeable and adaptable team.**
5. **B. Identifying and addressing inefficiencies in the verification process.**
6. **B. Gauging performance and identifying improvement areas.**
7. **B. Using metrics and data analysis to measure and improve effectiveness.**
8. **C. Generation of new ideas for process enhancement.**
9. **B. Prioritizing quality and shared responsibility for improvement.**

10. **C. Enhances the process through diverse perspectives and expertise.**

Chapter 15: The Future of Insurance Verification

15.1 Predicting Future Trends in Health Insurance

Predicting the future trends in health insurance and their impact on insurance verification is akin to charting a course in uncharted waters. The healthcare landscape is evolving rapidly, influenced by technological advancements, regulatory changes, and shifting patient expectations. Let's explore the potential future trends in health insurance and how they may shape the insurance verification processes.

Increased Use of Technology and Automation

- **Artificial Intelligence (AI):** AI is expected to play a more significant role in automating and streamlining insurance verification processes, reducing human error and improving efficiency.

- **Machine Learning:** Machine learning algorithms could predict common verification issues, allowing for proactive management of potential errors or denials.

Expansion of Telehealth Services

- **Telehealth Coverage:** As telehealth continues to grow, insurance policies are likely to adapt, providing more comprehensive coverage for remote healthcare services.

- **Verification Adjustments:** Insurance verification processes will need to adjust to cater to the nuances of telehealth services.

Enhanced Patient Engagement and Self-Service

- **Patient-Centric Models:** Insurance models are likely to become more patient-centric, with increased transparency and patient involvement in their care and coverage.

- **Self-Service Platforms:** The rise in self-service options, where patients can independently verify their insurance coverage, is anticipated to grow.

Changes in Healthcare Regulations

- **Regulatory Evolution:** Ongoing changes in healthcare laws and insurance regulations will require continuous adaptation in verification processes.

- **Compliance Focus:** Ensuring compliance with evolving regulations will remain a critical aspect of the insurance verification process.

Integration of Wearable Technology and Health Data

- **Data-Driven Coverage:** Wearable technology and health data analytics may influence insurance coverage decisions and personalized insurance plans.

- **Verification Complexity:** The integration of personal health data into insurance verification could add layers of complexity, requiring more advanced verification solutions.

Personalized Insurance Plans

- **Customized Coverage:** There may be a shift towards more personalized insurance plans based on individual health needs and lifestyles.

- **Adaptive Verification Processes:** Verification processes will need to adapt to handle the variances in personalized insurance plans.

Blockchain in Insurance Verification

- **Secure Data Management:** Blockchain technology could be utilized for secure and transparent handling of insurance data, enhancing integrity and reducing fraud.

- **Smart Contracts:** Blockchain might enable the implementation of smart contracts for automated verification and authorization.

Conclusion

The future of health insurance verification is poised to be deeply intertwined with technological advancements and regulatory changes. Staying agile, continuously embracing innovation, and adapting to new models of patient care and insurance will be essential for healthcare providers. By anticipating these trends, the healthcare industry can prepare for a future where insurance verification is more efficient, patient-focused, and technologically driven.

15.2 Preparing for Changes in Healthcare Legislation

Adapting to changes in healthcare legislation is a critical aspect of managing insurance verification, akin to navigating a ship through shifting tides. Healthcare laws and regulations are continually evolving, and staying compliant and informed is essential for the smooth operation of healthcare services. Let's explore how healthcare providers can prepare for these legislative changes.

Staying Informed

- **Regular Updates:** Keep abreast of legislative changes by subscribing to healthcare news, attending industry conferences, and participating in relevant webinars and seminars.

- **Engagement with Professional Associations:** Maintain active involvement with professional healthcare associations that provide insights and updates on legislative changes.

Staff Training and Development

- **Ongoing Education:** Regularly update training programs to reflect the latest healthcare laws and insurance regulations.

- **Specialized Training Sessions:** Conduct specialized training sessions to focus on significant legislative changes and their implications on insurance verification.

Policy Review and Adaptation

- **Internal Policy Updates:** Regularly review and update internal policies and procedures to ensure they align with the latest legislation.

- **Flexibility in Processes:** Develop verification processes that are flexible and can be quickly adjusted to accommodate new legislative requirements.

Risk Management

- **Risk Assessment:** Regularly assess the potential risks associated with legislative changes and how they might impact insurance verification.

- **Contingency Planning:** Develop contingency plans to address potential challenges or disruptions resulting from legislative changes.

Technology and System Upgrades

- **Software Compliance:** Ensure that the software systems used for insurance verification are up-to-date and compliant with the latest healthcare legislation.

- **System Flexibility:** Choose verification systems that are adaptable and can be easily updated to accommodate new legal requirements.

Collaboration and Communication

- **Insurance Company Partnerships:** Work closely with insurance companies to understand how legislative changes will affect their policies and, in turn, the verification process.

- **Clear Communication with Patients:** Keep patients informed about how legislative changes might affect their insurance coverage and verification processes.

Legal Consultation

- **Legal Expertise:** Engage with legal experts who specialize in healthcare law to get advice on complying with new regulations.

- **Regular Legal Audits:** Conduct audits with legal assistance to ensure continuous compliance with healthcare legislation.

Feedback Mechanism

- **Staff and Patient Feedback:** Encourage feedback from staff and patients regarding the implementation of new legislative changes to continually improve processes.

- **Monitoring Impact:** Monitor the impact of legislative changes on the verification process and patient experiences, making adjustments as necessary.

Conclusion

Preparing for changes in healthcare legislation is an ongoing process that requires vigilance, adaptability, and proactive planning. By staying informed, continuously training staff, updating policies, and utilizing flexible technology systems, healthcare providers can effectively navigate the changing legal landscape and maintain efficient and compliant insurance verification processes.

15.3 Embracing Technological Advancements

In the rapidly evolving field of healthcare, embracing technological advancements is critical for staying ahead in insurance verification. Technology not only enhances efficiency and accuracy but also offers new ways to manage and streamline the verification process. It's like equipping a ship with the latest navigation tools to voyage through the complex sea of healthcare insurance. Let's explore how embracing technological advancements can reshape insurance verification.

Artificial Intelligence and Machine Learning

- **Automated Verification:** AI can automate routine verification tasks, reducing manual workload and minimizing errors.

- **Predictive Analysis:** Machine learning algorithms can analyze historical data to predict common issues, enabling proactive management of verification challenges.

Blockchain Technology

- **Secure Data Management:** Blockchain can offer a secure and transparent way to manage patient insurance data, enhancing privacy and reducing fraud.

- **Smart Contracts:** Implement smart contracts in blockchain to automate certain aspects of insurance verification and authorization.

Cloud-Based Solutions

- **Accessibility and Collaboration:** Cloud-based platforms allow for easier access to insurance data, facilitating collaboration among different healthcare providers.

- **Real-Time Updates:** Utilize cloud services for real-time updates on insurance policies and patient coverage details.

Internet of Medical Things (IoMT) and Wearables

- **Integration with Patient Data:** IoMT devices and wearables can provide real-time health data, potentially influencing insurance verification and personalized insurance plans.

- **Enhanced Patient Engagement:** These technologies can engage patients more actively in their health management, impacting their insurance coverage and verification.

Advanced Analytics and Big Data

- **Data-Driven Decisions:** Use big data analytics to gain insights into insurance trends, patient demographics, and verification outcomes to inform strategic decisions.

- **Error Identification:** Analyze large sets of verification data to identify patterns in errors or denials, guiding process improvements.

Telehealth and Remote Verification

- **Adapting to Telehealth:** As telehealth services grow, develop systems for remote verification of insurance coverage, catering to the unique needs of virtual care.

- **Digital Communication Tools:** Utilize digital tools for patient-provider communication regarding insurance verification in a telehealth context.

Mobile Technology

- **Patient-Facing Apps:** Develop or utilize mobile applications that allow patients to submit their insurance information, check coverage details, and receive updates on verification status.

- **QR Code Scanning:** Use QR codes for quick and secure retrieval of patient insurance information.

Custom Software Development

- **Tailored Solutions:** Develop custom software solutions that cater specifically to the unique needs of your healthcare facility's verification processes.

- **Integration with Existing Systems:** Ensure that new software integrates seamlessly with existing electronic health records and billing systems.

Conclusion

Embracing technological advancements in insurance verification offers numerous opportunities to enhance efficiency, accuracy, and patient engagement. By leveraging AI, blockchain, cloud computing, IoMT, and other emerging technologies, healthcare providers can not only streamline the verification process but also adapt to the changing landscape of healthcare delivery and insurance.

15.4 Exercise: 10 MCQs with Answers at the End

1. **How does artificial intelligence (AI) impact insurance verification?**

   A. Increases manual workload.

   B. Reduces accuracy and efficiency.

   C. Automates routine tasks and reduces errors.

   D. Makes the process more complex.

2. **What role can blockchain technology play in insurance verification?**

   A. Decrease data security.

   B. Create more paperwork.

   C. Provide secure and transparent data management.

   D. Eliminate the need for verification.

3. **How do cloud-based solutions benefit insurance verification?**

A. Limit data accessibility.

B. Complicate collaboration among healthcare providers.

C. Allow for easier access to insurance data and facilitate collaboration.

D. Increase data vulnerability.

4. **What impact could Internet of Medical Things (IoMT) devices have on insurance verification?**

A. They are irrelevant to insurance processes.

B. Provide real-time health data influencing verification.

C. Decrease patient engagement.

D. Complicate the verification process unnecessarily.

5. **Why is big data analytics important in insurance verification?**

A. It has no significant impact.

B. For analyzing trends and improving decision-making.

C. To increase the error rate in verification.

D. To ignore patient data and trends.

6. **What advantage does mobile technology offer in insurance verification?**

A. Reduces patient involvement.

B. Makes the process less secure.

C. Allows patients to submit information and check coverage details via apps.

D. Increases the complexity for patients.

7. **How does custom software development benefit the insurance verification process?**

A. It is generally less effective than standard solutions.

B. Offers tailored solutions for specific verification needs.

C. Increases dependency on manual processes.

D. Slows down the verification process.

8. **What is a key benefit of using QR code technology in insurance verification?**

A. Slows down the information retrieval process.

B. Offers quick and secure retrieval of patient insurance information.

C. Complicates patient data entry.

D. Reduces data accuracy.

9. **How does telehealth impact insurance verification?**

A. Makes it obsolete.

B. Requires adaptations for remote verification.

C. Decreases the need for digital tools.

D. Simplifies all insurance policies.

10. **What is the significance of predictive analysis in insurance verification?**

A. It has no practical application.

B. Predicts common verification issues for proactive management.

C. Increases unpredictability in the process.

D. Focuses only on past data without influencing current processes.

Answers

1. **C. Automates routine tasks and reduces errors.**

2. **C. Provide secure and transparent data management.**

3. **C. Allow for easier access to insurance data and facilitate collaboration.**

4. **B. Provide real-time health data influencing verification.**

5. **B. For analyzing trends and improving decision-making.**

6. **C. Allows patients to submit information and check coverage details via apps.**

7. **B. Offers tailored solutions for specific verification needs.**

8. **B. Offers quick and secure retrieval of patient insurance information.**

9. **B. Requires adaptations for remote verification.**

10. **B. Predicts common verification issues for proactive management.**

Conclusion

As we conclude this comprehensive exploration of insurance verification in healthcare, it's evident that this area is both critical and complex, with far-reaching implications for healthcare providers, patients, and the overall healthcare system. The chapters we've covered provide a detailed insight into various aspects of insurance verification, from fundamental processes and compliance issues to advanced techniques and future trends.

Key takeaways from this exploration include:

1. **Importance of Accuracy and Efficiency:** Accurate and efficient insurance verification is essential for minimizing claim denials, ensuring financial stability for healthcare providers, and reducing patient stress and confusion.

2. **Evolving Landscape:** The insurance verification landscape is continuously evolving, influenced by changes in healthcare legislation, insurance policies, and technological advancements.

3. **Technological Integration:** Embracing modern technology, such as AI, blockchain, and cloud-based solutions, can significantly enhance the verification process, making it more efficient and accurate.

4. **Patient-Centric Approach:** As healthcare moves towards a more patient-centric model, transparency, clear communication, and patient education become increasingly important in the insurance verification process.

5. **Continuous Improvement:** Ongoing training, regular auditing, and a focus on continuous improvement are crucial for adapting to changes in the healthcare landscape and maintaining high standards in insurance verification.

6. **Future Trends:** Future trends, including the rise of telehealth, personalized insurance plans, and the integration of wearable technology, will continue to shape and redefine the processes and strategies in insurance verification.

7. **Preparation for Legislative Changes:** Staying informed and agile in response to healthcare legislation changes is critical for compliance and continued effectiveness in insurance verification.

8. **Collaboration and Communication:** Effective communication and collaboration with patients, insurance companies, and across healthcare departments are vital for a seamless verification process.

In conclusion, insurance verification is a dynamic and indispensable component of the healthcare system. By understanding its complexities, staying informed about current trends and future directions, and continuously striving for improvement and adaptation, healthcare providers can ensure effective insurance verification, leading to optimized operational efficiency, financial health, and enhanced patient care.

The best way to thank an author is to write a review.

9 789334 008098

Printed at Repro India Ltd.